A Colour Atlas of
HYPERTENSION

Presented by
B. C. Bracklehurst.

Kim M. Fox
MD MRCP
Consultant Cardiologist

Leonard M. Shapiro
MD MRCP
Senior Registrar

National Heart Hospital, London

Wolfe Medical Publications Limited

Copyright ©️ Kim M. Fox, Leonard M. Shapiro 1986
Published by Wolfe Medical Publications 1986
Printed by Royal Smeets Offset b.v., Weert, Netherlands
ISBN 0 7234 08629

This book is one of the titles in the series of
Wolfe Medical Atlases, a series which brings
together probably the world's largest systematic
published collection of diagnostic colour
photographs.
For a full list of Atlases in the series, plus
forthcoming titles and details of our surgical,
dental and veterinary Atlases, please write to
Wolfe Medical Publications Ltd, Wolfe House,
3 Conway Street, London W1P 6HE.

General Editor, Wolfe Medical Atlases:
G. Barry Carruthers, MD(London)

Preface

Hypertension is the single most frequent disease in man, affecting up to 30% of the population. It is a multi-system disorder affecting the heart, kidney, brain and eye. In addition, rare endocrine disorders may present with hypertension. Hypertension is therefore of interest to any physician involved in clinical medicine.

This atlas is designed to illustrate the important clinical causes and effects of hypertension. The book is largely based on pathology which is shown together with the results of clinical investigations.

In general we feel that all the topics are adequately covered, obviously the selection must be personal and our own interest in cardiology will be apparent. We have also included techniques that although not widely available at present may well become so in the future, for example magnetic resonance and digital subtraction angiography.

It is hoped that this book will provide a better understanding of a common multi-system disorder.

Acknowledgements

We are indebted to the many friends and colleagues who contributed illustrations for this text. In particular, we acknowledge the help of Dr R. Donaldson who not ony provided illustrations but also advised us on the production of this atlas. We also wish to thank the following, who have lent us many illustrations; Dr M. Rapheal, Dr E. Olsen, Dr P. Crean, Dr Donald Longmore, Dr Richard Underwood, and Miss Caroline Westgate. The help of Miss Kathy Back in typing the text is gratefully acknowledged.

The authors are also grateful to the following for permission to use pictures from their colour atlases already published by Wolfe Medical Publications.

From *A Colour Atlas of Cardiac Pathology*
Geoffrey Farrer-Brown
Figures **8**, page 52; **1**, page 58; **2**, page 59; **1** and **2**, page 74; **3** and **4**, page 75; **26**, page 86; **27–30**, page 87; **31** and **32**, page 88; **61**, page 103; **69**, page 107

From *A Colour Atlas of Endocrinology*
R. Hall, D. Evered and R. Greene
Figures **1–3**, page 39; **7** and **8**, page 40; **11** and **14**, page 42; **15**, page 43; **21** and **22**, page 45

From *A Colour Atlas of the Eye and Systemic Disease* Erna E. Kritzinger and Barry E. Wright
Figures **36** and **37**, page 28

From *A Colour Atlas of General Pathology*
G. Austin Gresham
Figures **1** and **2**, page 114

From *A Colour Atlas of Geriatric Medicine*
Asif Kamal and J. C. Brocklehurst
Figures **1**, page 131; **2**, page 132

From *A Colour Atlas of Neuropathology*
C. S. Treip
Figure **3**, page 133

From *A Colour Atlas of Renal Diseases*
George Williams
Figures **2**, page 17; **3–5**, page 18; **6–8**, page 19; **10**, page 19; **11**, page 20; **12**, page 20; **14–17**, page 21; **28** and **29**, page 26; **33–35**, page 28; **38** and **39**, page 29; **43**, page 30; **52**, page 34; **54** and **55**, page 35; **1** and **2**, page 49; **1**, page 128

From *A Colour Atlas of Surgical Pathology*
W. Guthrie and R. Fawkes
Figures **22**, page 24; **24**, page 24; **47**, page 32; **51**, page 34; **4**, page 39; **5** and **6**, page 40; **12** and **13**, page 42; **20**, page 45

CONTENTS

CLINICAL ASSESSMENT OF HYPERTENSION

KOROTKOFF SOUNDS 1

I Abrupt sharp sound as pressure is reduced to just below systolic pressure.

II Prolonged, louder murmuring sound.

III Good clear sound with only a slight murmer.

IV Abrupt muffling of sound.

V Disappearance of sounds.

1 Korotkoff sounds. The systolic blood pressure is taken as korotkoff sound number one and the diastolic pressure is taken as korotkoff number five.

SOURCES OF ERROR IN TAKING THE BLOOD PRESSURE 2

1. Inaccurate sphygmomanometer including the zero point.

2. Spasm of the brachial artery due to rapid deflation.

3. Inadequate positioning of the cuff.

4. Wrong size of cuff.

5. Brachial artery calcification may result in falsely high blood pressure.

2 Sources of error in taking the blood pressure.

BLOOD PRESSURE DIFFERENCES IN THE ARMS 3

1. 20% of patients will have different arm blood pressure if taken separately.

2. Greatest normal difference in blood pressure in arms tends to occur in hypertensive patients.

3. If blood pressure is higher in one arm, suspect:
   (a) Supravalvular aortic stenosis.
   (b) Arterial obstruction.
   (c) Subclavian steal.

3 Blood pressure differences in the arms.

BLOOD PRESSURE MEASUREMENT IN THE LEGS 4

1. Blood pressure in the legs may be up to 20 mmHg more than arms.

2. Larger cuff must be used than the arm cuff.

3. Measure over popliteal artery with cuff on the thigh.

4. In children, doppler ultrasound is the method of choice.

4 Blood pressure measurement in the legs.

CLINICAL EXAMINATION OF THE HYPERTENSIVE PATIENT

A. *General*
1. Fundi.

2. Pulses.

3. Apex for left ventricular hypertrophy.

4. Heart sounds.

B. *Effects*
Examine for evidence of:
1. Cerebro-vascular disease.

2. Peripheral vascular disease.

3. Cardiac involvement including coronary disease, heart failure, aortic regurgitation and dissecting aneurysm.

4. Renal disease.

C. *Causes*
Examine for evidence of:
1. Renal causes especially renal artery stenosis, pyelo-nephritis, glomerulo-nephritis and diabetes.

2. Endocrine causes especially phaeochromocytoma, Cushing's and acromegaly.

3. Coarctation of the aorta.

5 Scheme for the clinical examination of a hypertensive patient.

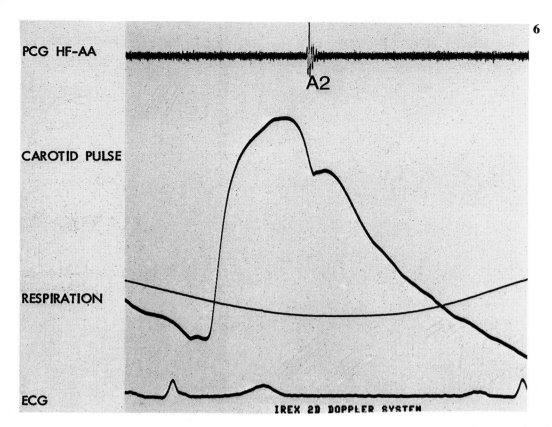

PCG HF-AA

A2

CAROTID PULSE

RESPIRATION

ECG

IREX 2D DOPPLER SYSTEM

6   The carotid pulse in a hyper-tensive subject. When examining the pulse it is important to be aware of the character of the pulse as well as the rhythm and whether all the pulses are full volume. Loud aortic closure will be heard and recorded on the phonocardiogram. PCG HF-AA – phonocardiogram high frequency aortic area.

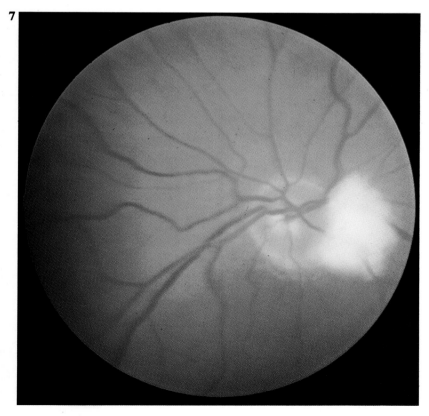

7   Normal optic fundus. There are medullated fibres seen in this normal fundus.

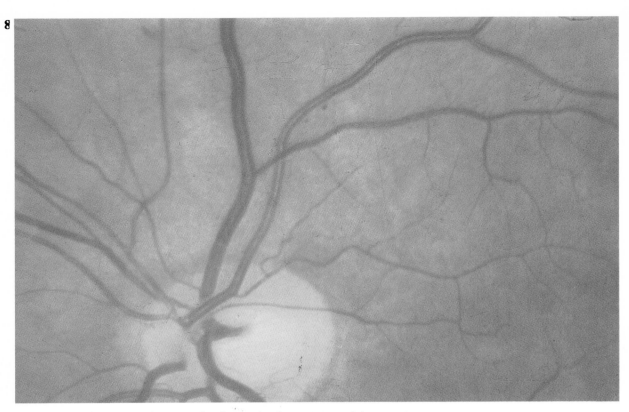

8   Grade 1 changes in the optic fundus with silver wiring of the arteries.

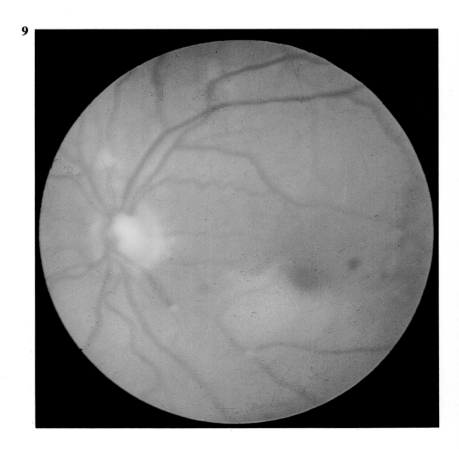

9   Grade three fundus with
haemorrhages and exudates.

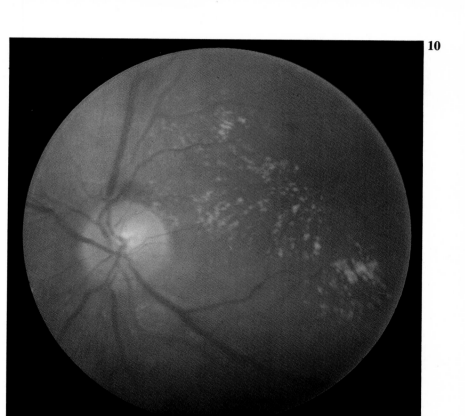

10 Grade three fundus with an extensive area of exudates.

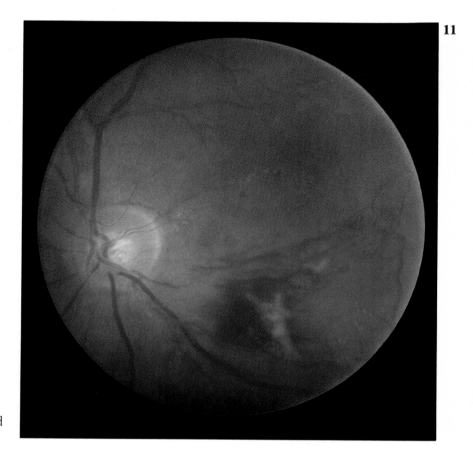

11 Grade three fundus with extensive areas of flame shaped haemorrhages.

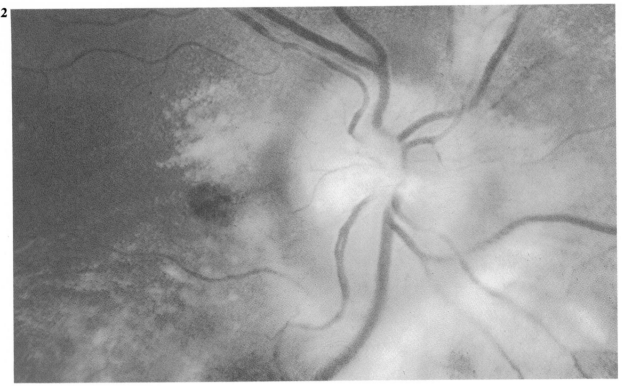

12 Grade four fundus with papilloedema and haemorrhage.

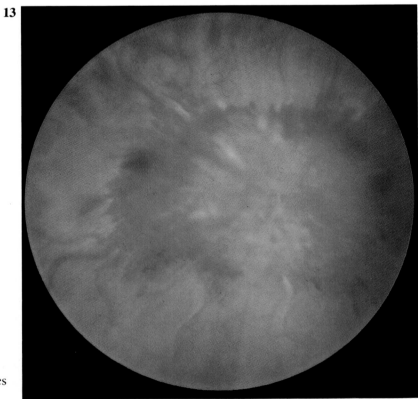

13 Severe grade four fundus with papilloedema, haemorrhages and exudates.

The Causes Of Hypertension

Approximately 5% of the middle aged population of Western countries have a diastolic blood pressure in excess of 110mmHg and a further 35% exceed 90mmHg (see **A**).

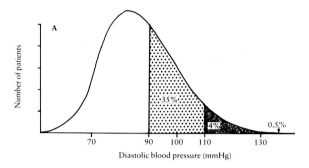

Normally diastolic pressure in the west rises with age and is greater in black males and females than in whites (see **B**).

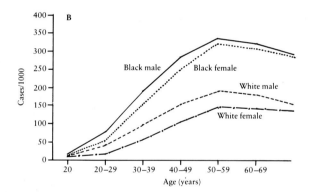

Factors known to influence blood pressure include family history and obesity, alcohol, smoking, salt intake and the oral contraceptive pill.

In more than 90% of patients with hypertension, the cause is unknown (primary or essential hypertension). Known causes of hypertension include renal disease, renovascular disease, endocrine abnormalities and coarctation of the aorta (see **C**).

The decision to investigate an individual patient will depend upon the age, sex, clinical signs, symptoms and severity of hypertension. At the initial clinical examination clues should be sought for underlying causes, thus aortic coarctation and Cushing's syndrome should be easily identified. A history of sweating,

pallor and palpitations should suggest phaeochromocytoma; butterfly skin rash on the face might raise the possibility of systemic lupus erythematosus. An abdominal bruit may be due to renal artery stenosis. A peripheral neuropathy would suggest diabetes.

Routine investigations performed to identify and quantify target organ damage may help to provide clues to underlying causes. Evidence of renal damage, eg elevated creatinine or proteinuria may be due to longstanding damage from essential hypertension, but should also raise the possiblity of underlying renal disease. The urine should be examined for glucose to exclude diabetes and an intravenous pyelogram will be necessary if there is any suspicion of an underlying renal cause. If it is thought that the renal disease is unilateral and, therefore, the possibility of a surgical cure is raised, renal venous renin ratios will need to be undertaken and an arteriogram performed to identify reno-vascular disease. Rarely, pyelonephritis is unilateral in which case if surgery is contemplated this must be confirmed by performing ureteric collections. If renal disease is bilateral, hypertension must be managed medically and further investigation will depend on the nature and severity of the renal abnormalities.

Renal artery stenosis may be treated surgically or by balloon angioplasty. Renal artery stenosis should be suspected if there is a sudden worsening of established hypertension

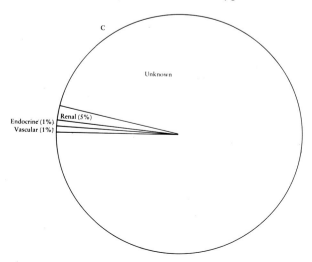

or in someone with previously documented normal blood pressure, or in hypertension occurring in the young, i.e. under the age of twenty years, or if there is a vascular bruit over the renal artery. Intravenous urograms will often show a delay in the first appearance of the contrast on the side of the stenosis, but even when investigation is very carefully undertaken, 20% of cases may be missed. Secretion of renin by the affected kidney will provide further evidence, but eventually arteriography will be necessary to accurately define the lesion.

Coarctation of the aorta is usually evident on clinical examination (radio-femoral delay, bruits over the back due to collaterals) and chest x-ray. If surgery is considered then arteriography will be necessary to define the lesion accurately.

Although responsible for less than 1% of cases of hypertension, an aldosterone producing adenoma produces a characteristic syndrome which is readily diagnosed and surgically curable. The tumour is almost always benign and solitary. Aldosterone causes sodium to be absorbed in the distal renal tubule with loss of potassium and hydrogen ions with progressive hypokalaemic alkalosis. The extent of the positive sodium balance is limited by proximal renal tubular escape as the plasma volume expands. Hypokalaemic alkalosis is usually asymptomatic, but when severe causes muscle weakness and even paralysis. The diagnosis of primary aldosteronism includes the demonstration of renin suppression, evidence of autonomous over secretion of aldosterone and finally localisation of the tumour by inferior vena cava and adrenal vein aldosterone levels.

Phaeochromocytomas are rare (0.1% of hypertensive subjects). They arise in sympathetic ganglia and they are usually benign, solitary adreno-medullary tumours but can be extramedullary and multiple. Phaeochromocytomas secrete varying proportions of noradrenaline, adrenaline, dopamine and other catecholamine precursors and metabolites. These have varying vasoconstrictor, vasodilator, cardioacceleratory and arrhythmogenic actions possibly causing hypertension (episodic, sustained, or sustained with episodic paroxysms), hypotension, tachycardia, bradycardia and arrhythmias. Excess noradrenaline and adrenaline stimulates sweating. Firm diagnosis is difficult, but 24-hour VMA levels, plasma adrenaline or noradrenaline and localisation by CT scanning should be performed. If intravenous urograms and venous sampling is undertaken, it is essential to pre-treat the patient with alpha and beta blocking agents.

Hypertension may be present in patients with Cushing's syndrome, but varies in severity. The patient usually presents for reasons other than hypertension and may have a typical appearance (overweight, moon face, striae, bruises, muscle weakness etc). Diagnosis is by measurement of adrenal steroids and ACTH, measured basally and following dexamethasone suppression and CT scanning of the adrenal gland and if appropriate the pituitary.

ESSENTIAL HYPERTENSION

> **1**
>
> Blood pressure = cardiac output × peripheral vascular resistance

1 Blood pressure is determined by a complex interplay of cardiac output and peripheral vascular resistance.

> **2**
>
> **INCREASED CARDIAC OUTPUT**
> 1. Left ventricular factors
> 2. Fluid load $\begin{cases} \text{Mineralocorticoids} \\ \text{Sodium loading} \end{cases}$

2 Elevation of either the cardiac output or the peripheral vascular resistance may lead to hypertension. This table shows the causes of increased cardiac output.

> **3**
>
> **INCREASED PERIPHERAL VASCULAR RESISTANCE**
> 1. Humoral, angiotensin and catecholamines
> 2. Sympathetic nervous system

3 This table shows the causes of increased peripheral vascular resistance.

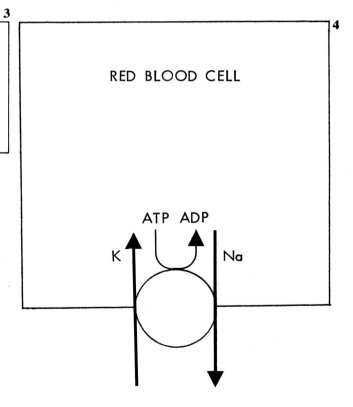

4 The role of dietary salt and the development of essential hypertension may be mediated by a familial abnormality of red blood cell cation transport as increased activity of the ouabain sensitive sodium-potassium-ATPase system.

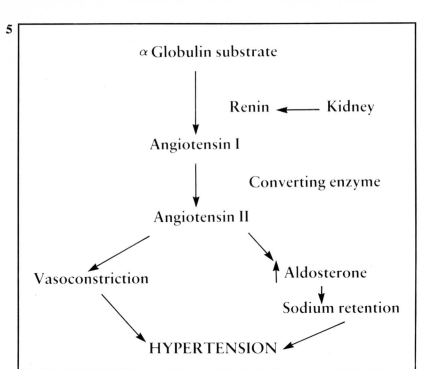

5 The role of the renin-angiotensin-aldosterone system is well documented in renovascular hypertension. Its importance in essential hypertension is less important, but plasma-renin activity is raised in 10% of patients.

6

Alcohol

Stress?

Polycythaemia

Oral contraceptives

Diabetes mellitus

Gout

Obesity

6 Other factors that may be important in the development of essential hypertension are shown here.

RENAL CAUSES OF HYPERTENSION

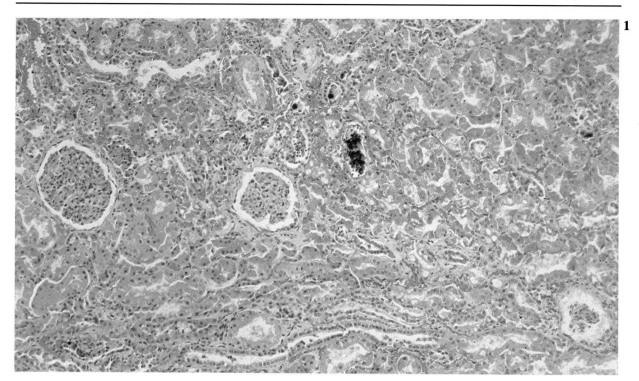

1 Histological haemotoxylin and eosin sections showing a normal glomerulus and tubules.

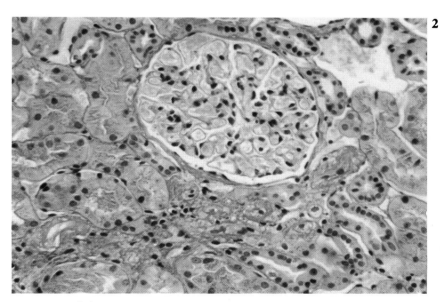

2 Minimal change type glomerulo-nephritis. No structural change is detected in this glomerulo-corpuscle by light microscopy.

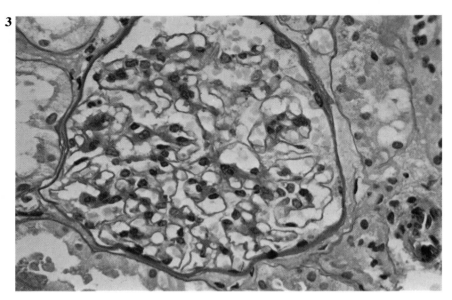

3 Histological section showing minimal change type glomerulo-nephritis. There is slight prominence of mesangial cells, b no other detected abnormality. Capillary basement membranes are of normal thickness (PAS × 512).

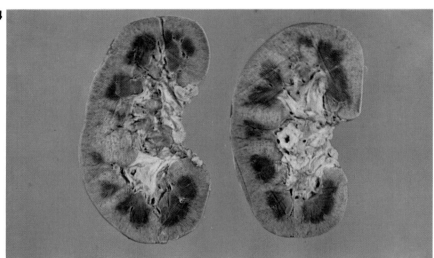

4 Macroscopic sections of kidne showing idiopathic membranous glomerulo-nephritis. The kidney enlarged and on section shows a characteristic pallor of its cortex contrast with the darker medulla

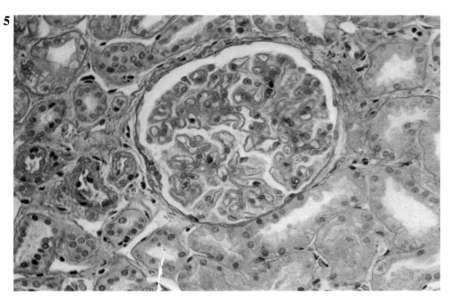

5 Histological section showing idiopathic membranous glomerulo-nephritis. The main abnormality is the uniform thickening of the capillary basement membranes (MSB × 224).

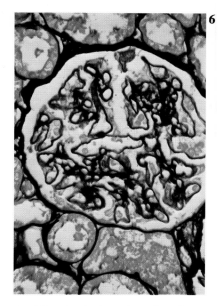

6 Histological section showing basement membrane thickening with the sections stained with silver (MeS × 330).

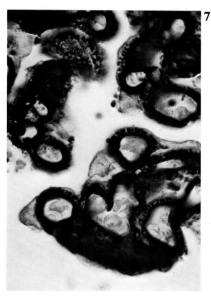

7 Histological section showing idiopathic membranous glomerulo-nephritis. Thicker section of glomerulo-capillary loop shows thickened basement membranes with characteristic spike projections along their epimembranous borders (MeS × 1496).

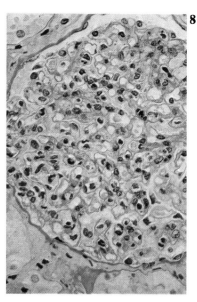

8 Histological section showing increased cellularity of glomerulus in acute proliferative glomerulo-nephritis. There are occasional polymorph leucocytes in capillary lumena (PAS × 330).

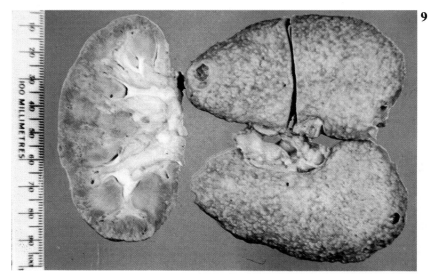

9 Macroscopic section showing slowly progressive phase of diffuse glomerulo-nephritis. There is reduction of parenchyma particularly of the cortex with increase in peri-pelvic fat content. The sub-capsular surface is granular with cyst formation at one pole.

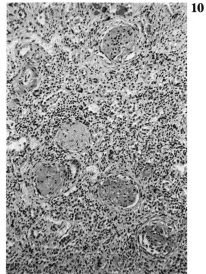

10 Histological section from the kidney shown in 9.
There is hyalinisation of the glomeruli (some of which show capsular adhesions) and severe atrophy of tubules. The interstitium shows diffuse lymphocytic infiltration (H and E × 132).

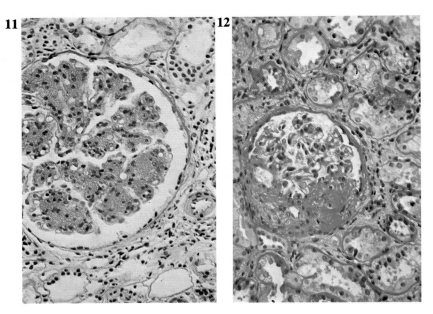

11 Histological section showing chronic lobular glomerulo-nephritis. There is pronounced lobulation of the glomerular tufts with excess of hyaline mesangial matrix (PAS × 330).

12 Histological section showing focal proliferative glomerulo-nephritis with cellular proliferation and hyalinisation in lower glomerular lobules (PAS × 330).

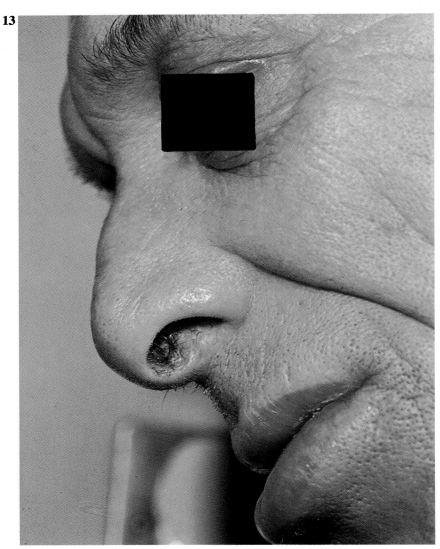

13 Clinical appearance in acute glomerulo-nephritis with oedema characteristically involving the face.

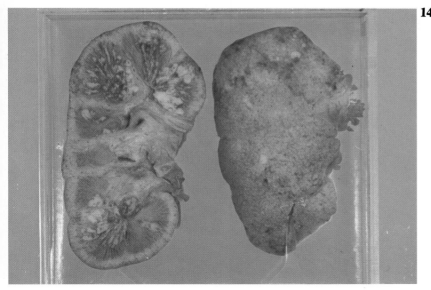

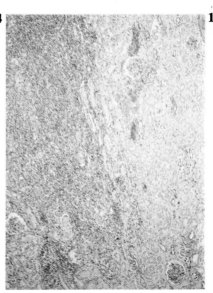

14 Macroscopic section showing acute pyelo-nephritis; haemorrhagic areas are surrounded by multiple abscesses.

15 Microscopic section showing acute pyelo-nephritis with areas of acute interstitial inflammation (H and E × 352).

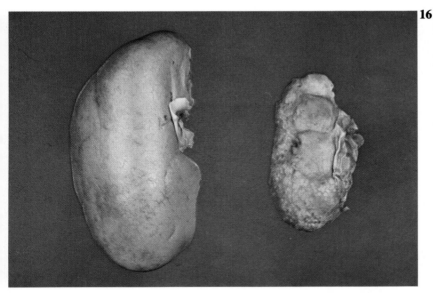

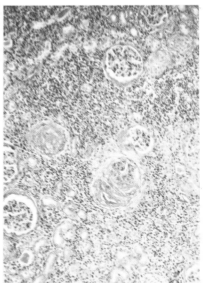

16 Macroscopic section showing chronic pyelo-nephritis. Normal kidney (left) contrasts with severely scarred contracted kidney of chronic pyelo-nephritis (right).

17 Microscopic section showing chronic pyelo-nephritis with dense interstitial inflammation, sclerosis of glomeruli and loss of tubules (MSB × 143).

18

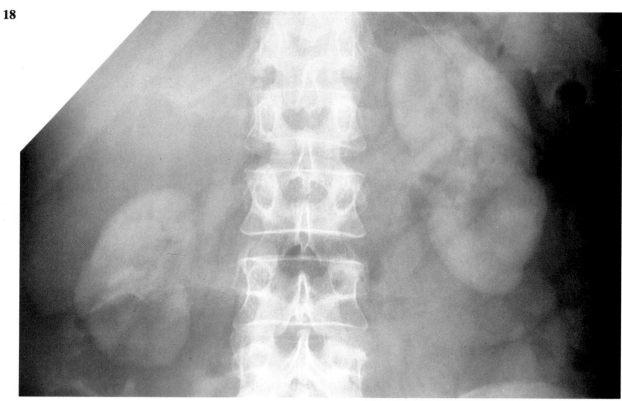

18   Intravenous urogram of chronic pyelo-nephritis. This shows a deformed and shrunken right kidney.

19

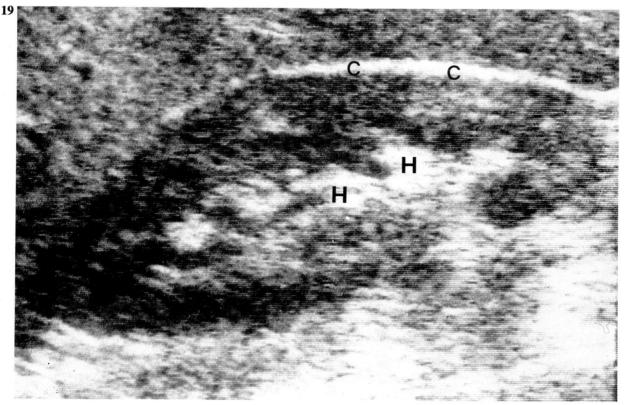

19   Normal renal ultrasound. Showing the renal capsule (C) and hilium (H).

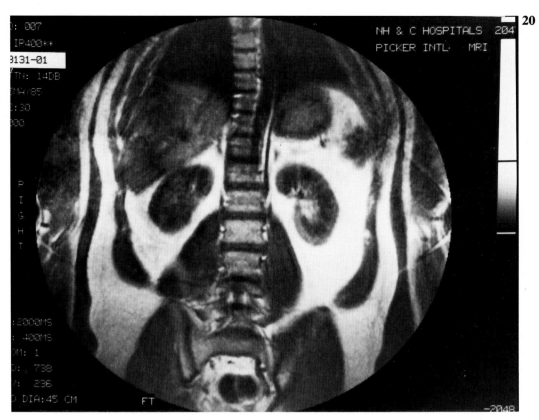

20 Magnetic resonance scan in coronal section showing the normal kidneys.

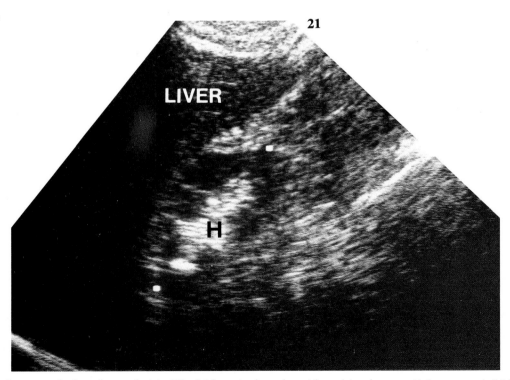

21 Ultrasound of pyelo-nephritis. The kidney is shrunken (the white dots are 7.5cm apart). H-hilum.

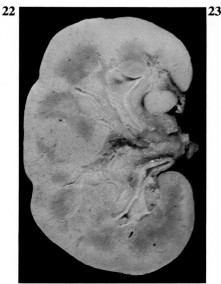

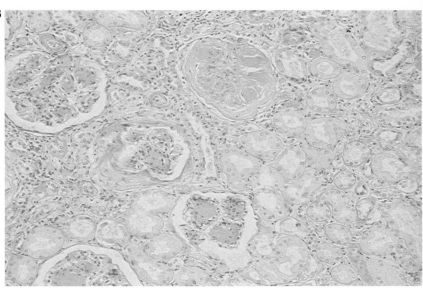

22 Macroscopic section showing diabetic kidney with granulomatous ureteritis.

23 Histological section at low power showing Kimmelstiel-Wilson nodular glomerulo-sclerosis (H and E stain).

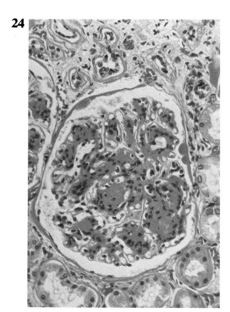

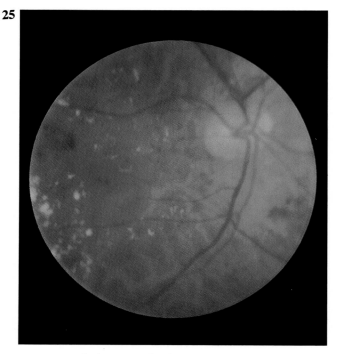

24 Histological section showing Kimmelstiel-Wilson nodular glomerulo-sclerosis and lozenges on Bowman's capsule at higher power (H and E × 83).

25 Retinal photograph of patient with insulin dependent diabetes. This shows cotton-wool spots and microaneurysms. Background retinopathy is frequently associated with the early stages of diabetic renal disease.

26 Retinal photography of an insulin dependent diabetic with proliferative retinopathy. There are areas of new vessel formation and extensive haemorrhages. The patient has undergone photocoagulation. Such patients almost always have diabetic renal disease and this is frequently associated with hypertension. It would appear that hypertension accelerates the development of diabetic proliferative retinopathy.

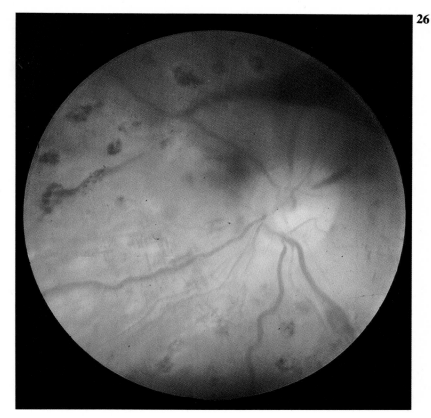

27 Combination of malignant hypertension and diabetic proliferative retinopathy.

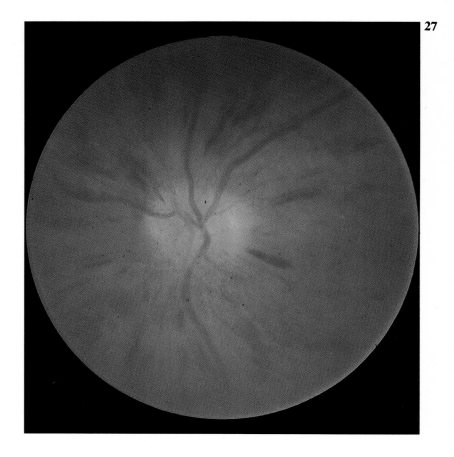

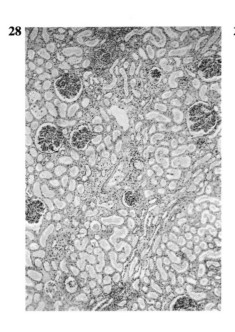 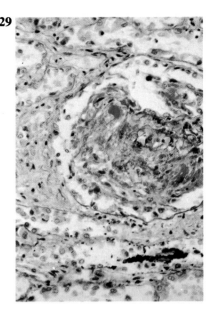

28 Histology showing polyarteritis nodosa in the acute phase. Glomeruli are diffusely hypercellular. Fibrinoid foci are difficult to identify at low magnification (H and E × 55).

29 Histology showing disruption of glomerular structure produced by proliferative change and fibrinoid necrosis in acute polyarteritis nodosa (MSB × 330).

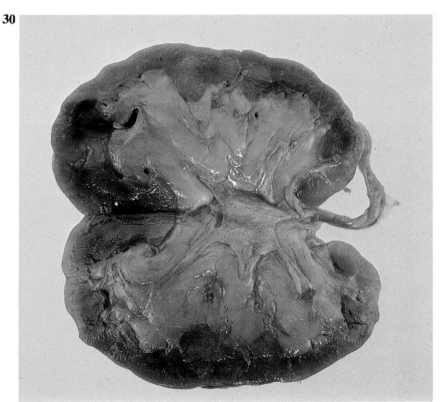

30 Macroscopic view of the kidney showing areas of infarction in a patient with polyarteritis nodosa.

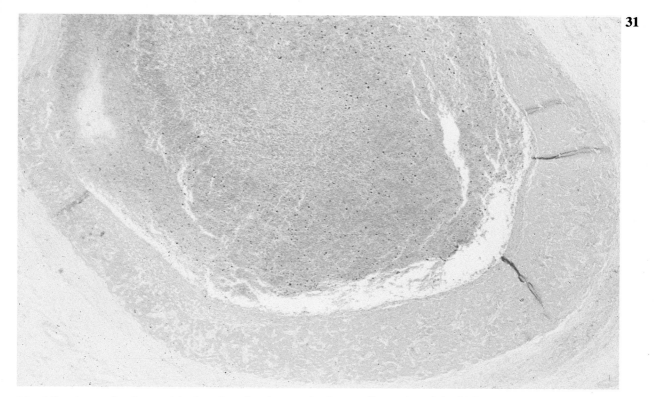

31 Histology of polyarteritis showing the changes in the small arteries of the kidneys.

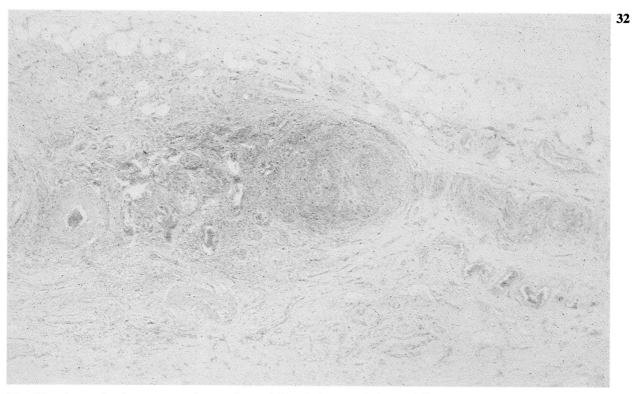

32 Histology of polyarteritis. Glomeruli are diffusely hypercellular and fibrinoid foci may be seen.

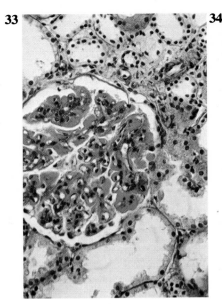

33 Histology showing widespread fibrinoid involvement of the glomerular capillaries in systemic lupus erythematosus (MSB × 330).

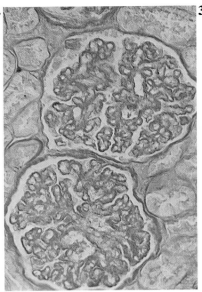

34 Histology of systemic lupus erythematosis showing characteristic wireloop lesion of glomerular capillaries producing a uniform thickening of the basement membrane (PAS × 286).

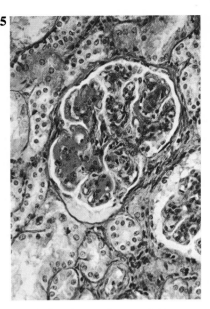

35 Histology of necrotising glomerulo-nephritis in systemic lupus erythematosis shown as fibrinoid (red) necrosis of capillary loops and focal cellular damage (MSB × 330).

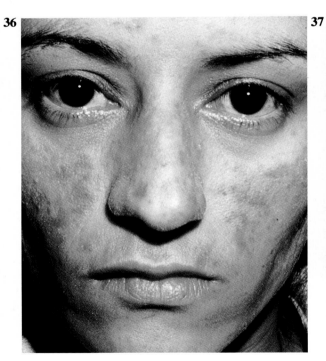

36 An erythematous butterfly rash on the face is a classic sign of systemic lupus erythematosus.

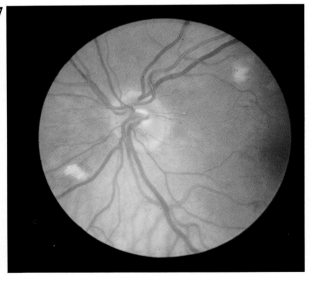

37 Cotton-wool spots in the fundus. These are caused by localised infarction of the retinal nerve fibre layer and reflect severe retinal ischaemia.

38 Macroscopic section of a hemisected kidney in systemic sclerosis showing normal kidney size but cortex is diffusely mottled and contains several minute infarcts.

39 Histology showing fibrinoid necrosis extending into glomerular capillaries in systemic sclerosis (MSB × 308).

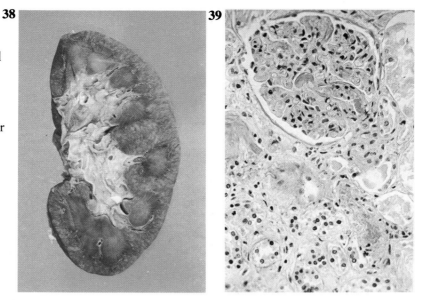

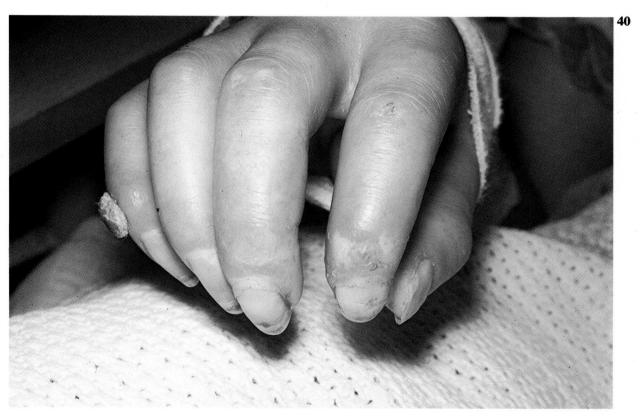

40 The hand in systemic sclerosis showing thickening and tightening of the skin particularly around the fingers. There are also calcium deposits around the finger-tips.

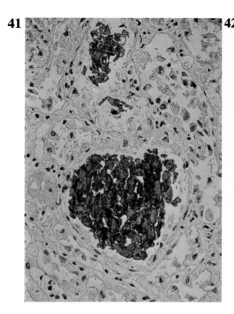 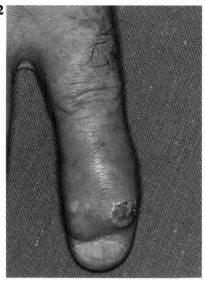

41 Histology in renal gout. The urate crystals give a positive (grey/green) Schultz reaction (Shultz × 330).

42 This shows a gouty tophus in the finger.

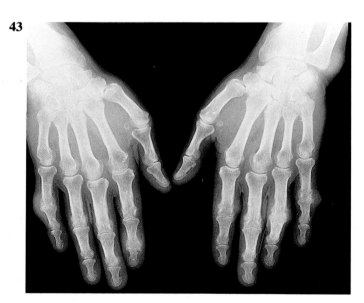

43 X-ray of the hands in a patient with gout. There is soft-tissue swelling and bony erosions.

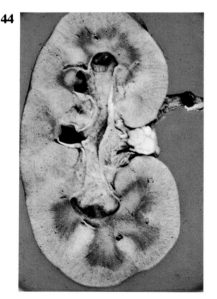

44 Macroscopic section showing renal amyloidosis. Hemisected kidney showing characteristic wide pale cortex.

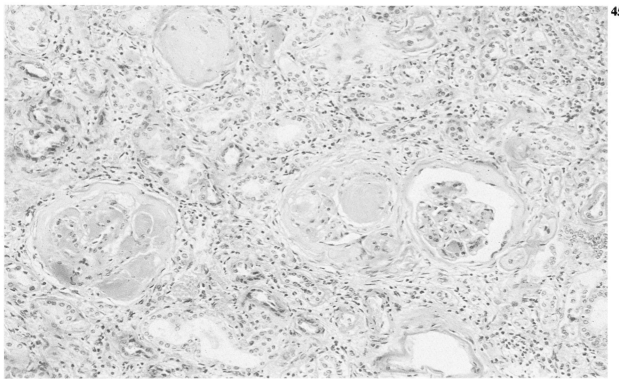

45 Microscopic section showing amyloid infiltration of glomerular capillaries producing thickened basement membranes.

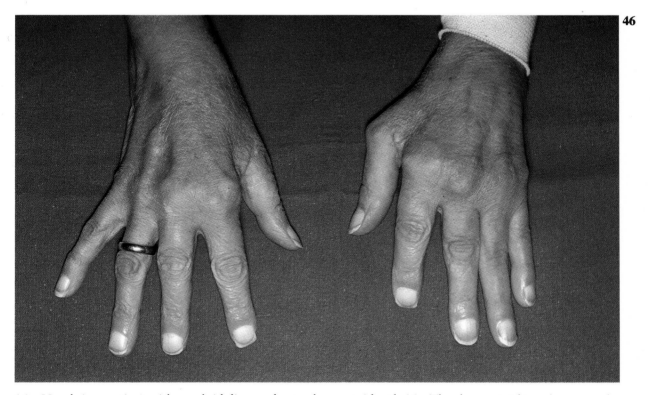

46 Hands in a patient with amyloid disease due to rheumatoid arthritis. The rheumatoid involvement of the fingers of the hand can be clearly seen.

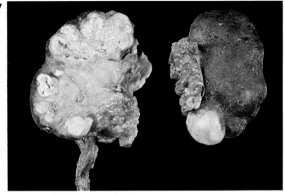

47 Macroscopic section showing tuberculosis of the kidney and ureter. The outer surface of the kidney appears lobulated, one dilated calyx appearing white at one pole is also seen. The cut surface shows pieces of material replacing nearly all of the parenchyma and areas of calcification.

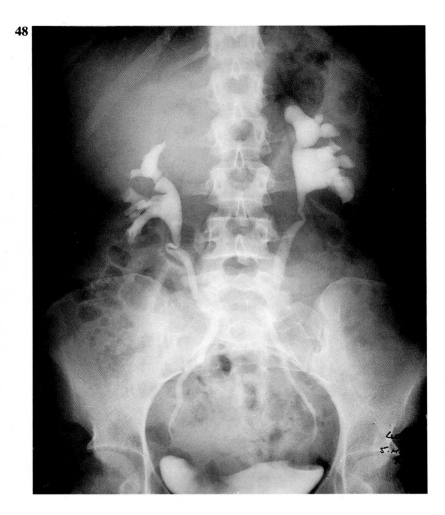

48 Intravenous urogram of tuberculous kidney showing dilated and deformed pelvicalyceal system.

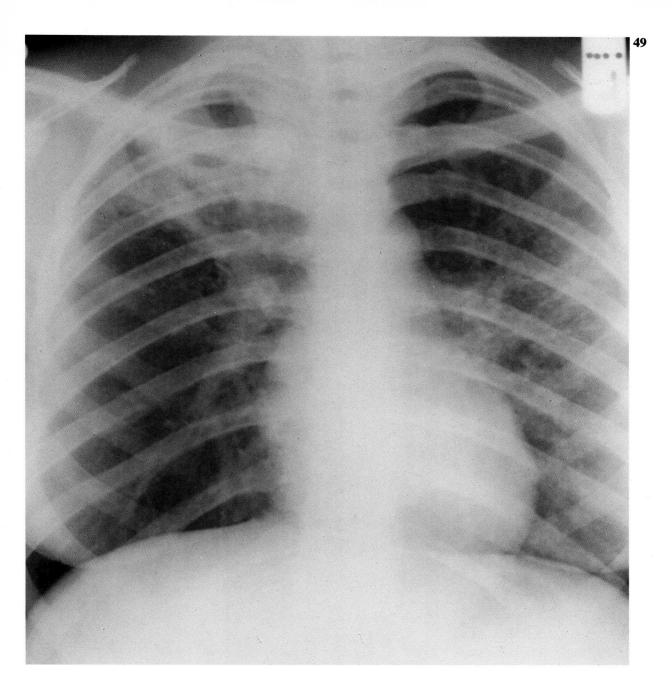

49 Chest x-ray in tuberculosis in the same patient as **48**, showing fibrosis with a cavity in the right upper lobe.

50

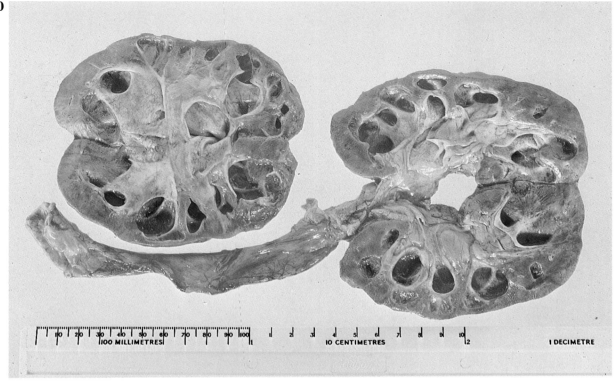

50   Hydronephrosis of the kidney. The dilated pelvicalyceal system is clearly seen as is the thin cortex and medulla.

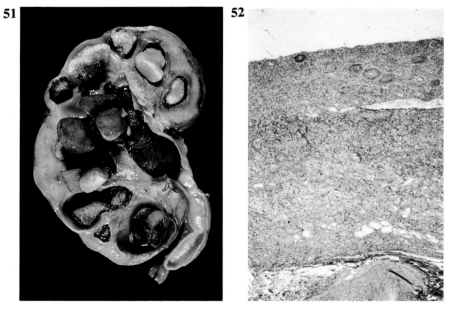

51

52

51   Macroscopic section of chronic pyelo-nephritis and hydronephrosis with staghorn calculus. The dilated pelvis is filled with calculus and the cortex is paper-thin in places. There were two stenoses in the proximal ureter which is dilated.

52   Microscopic section of severe hydronephrosis showing atrophy of nephrons and glomerulo-sclerosis (MSB × 66).

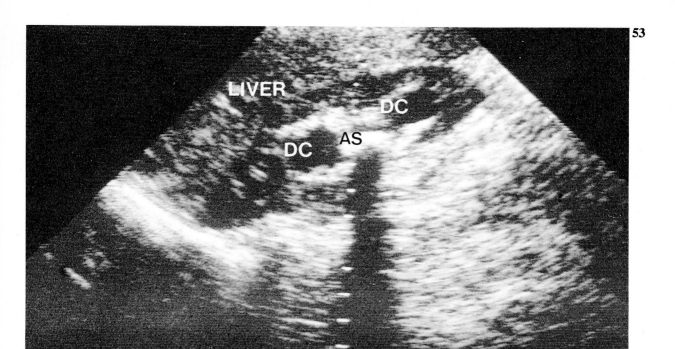

53 Ultrasound of hydronephrosis. The calyxes are dilated (DC) and an acoustic shadow (AS) corresponds to a renal calculus.

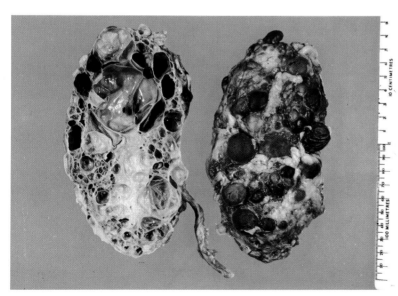

54 Macroscopic views of the kidneys showing polycystic disease. Both surfaces show masses of thin wall cysts.

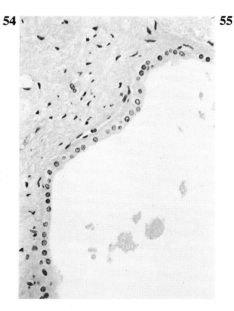

55 Microscopic section of polycystic disease. Cyst walls are formed of connective tissue with low cuboidal epithelium (H and E × 330).

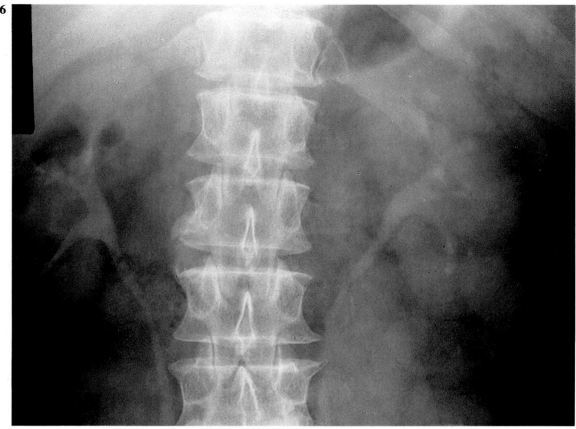

56   Intravenous urogram of polycystic disease showing large kidneys with cysts indenting the renal collecting system.

57

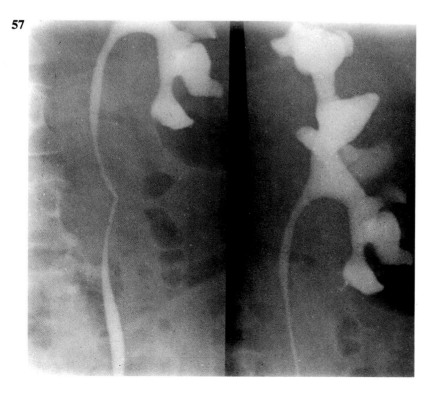

57   Retrograde urogram in polycystic disease with gross deformity of the pelvicalyceal system.

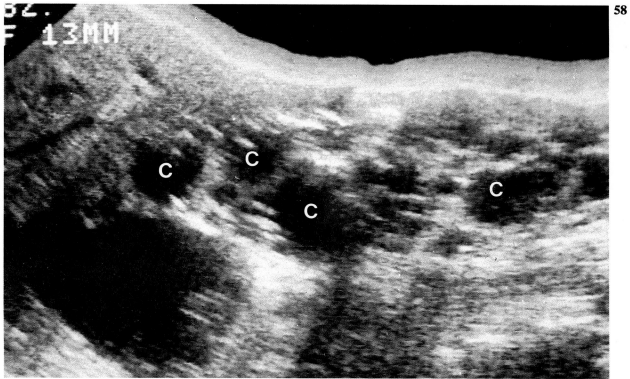

58 Renal ultrasound of polycystic disease. Large polycystic kidney (20 cm) with multiple cysts (C) of different sizes.

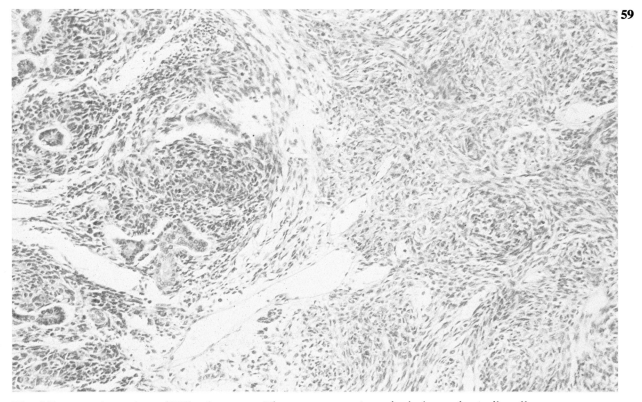

59 Microscopic section of Wilms' tumour. The tumour consists of tubular and spindle cell components.

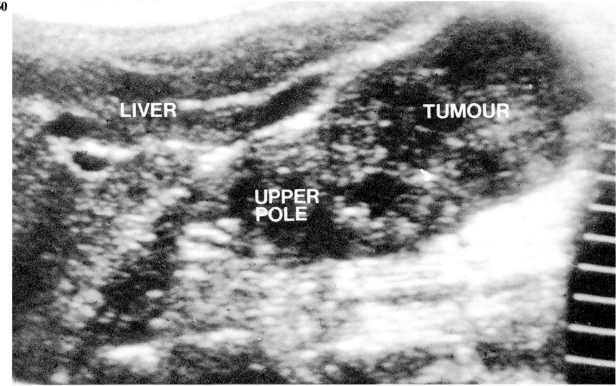

60 Ultrasound of Wilms' tumour. The tumour occupies the upper pole of the right kidney.

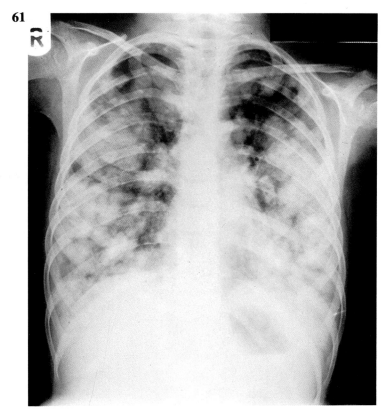

61 Chest x-ray showing multiple metastases in a patient with Wilms' tumour.

ENDOCRINE CAUSES OF HYPERTENSION

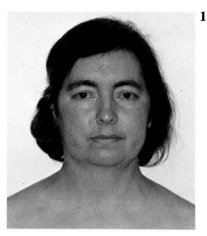

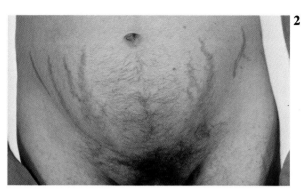

2 Purple striae on the abdomen of a patient with Cushing's syndrome. There is characteristic thinning of the skin.

1 Patient with Cushinoid appearance to the face. The most striking features are rounding of the face, hirsutism, loss of hair, acne and pigmentation.

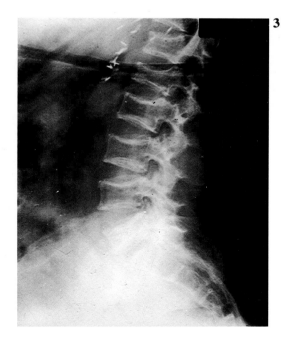

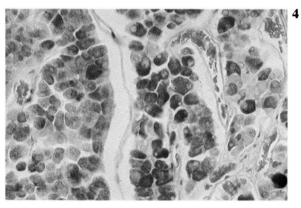

4 Basophil adenoma of the pituitary gland from a 58-year-old woman who was hypertensive, clinically regarded as having Cushing's syndrome.

3 Osteoporosis is a major feature of Cushing's syndrome and may lead to loss of height and pathological fractures. The features seen in **1** and **2**, this page will also occur secondary to cortico-steroid treatment.

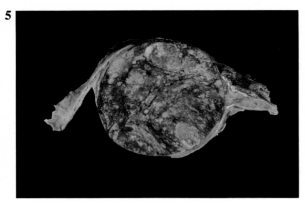

5   Cortical adenoma (brown tumour) of the adrenal glands. This was taken from a 49-year-old man with Cushing's syndrome who presented with hypertension, osteoporosis, generalised weakness and a moon face. The adenoma has a dark brown and yellow cut surface.

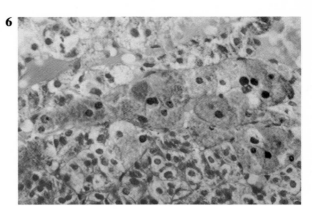

6   Histological specimen of cortical adenoma from 5. This shows that there are three types of cell (× 330).

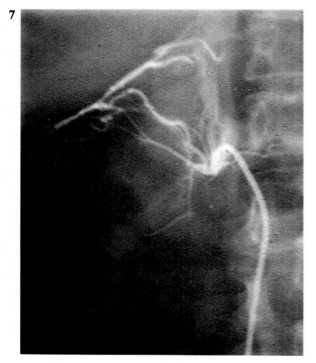

7   Selective venogram of adrenal tumour.

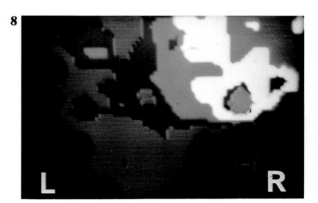

8   Labelled cholesterol scan showing a right adrenal tumour in a patient with Cushing's syndrome.

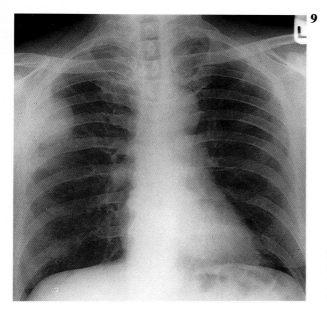

9 Solitary lesion in chest x-ray. Such lesions may lead to the ectopic ACTH syndrome. The patient presented with a Cushinoid type appearance.

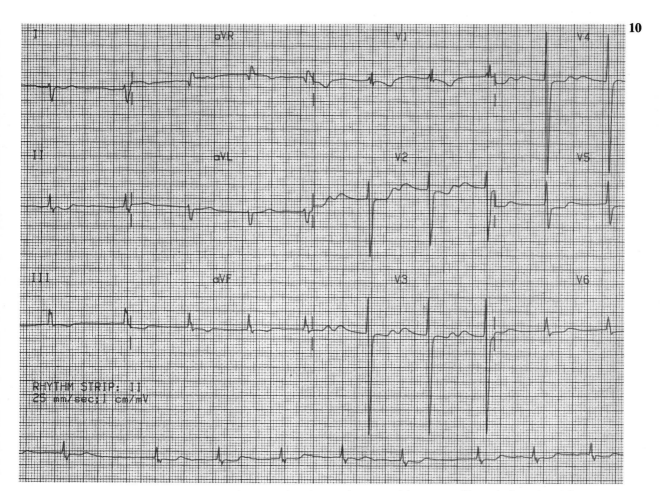

10 Electrocardiogram in Conn's syndrome. This shows the typical features of hypokalaemia with a significant U wave, ST depression, T wave inversion and prolonged QT.

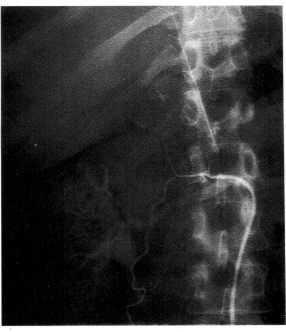

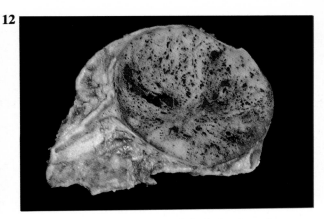

12 Phaeochromocytoma of the left adrenal gland. This specimen is from a 37-year-old man with paroxysmal hypertension.

11 Conn's syndrome. This is a very rare cause of hypertension. The characteristic biochemical abnormalities are hypernatraemia, hypokalaemia and suppression of renal production. These may arise from renal tumours or hyperplasia of the zona glomerulosa. These adrenal tumours may be very small, but can generally be demonstrated by angiography.

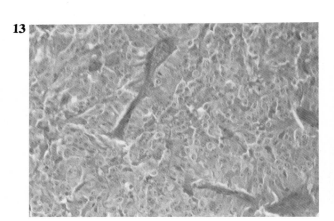

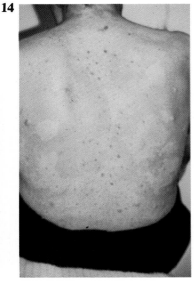

13 Phaeochromocytoma. Same example as in **12**, this page. This section shows the alveolar arrangement of polyhedral cells resembling those of the normal medulla. They have abundant eosinophilic cytoplasm with refined pigment granules giving a positive reaction after chrome fixation (H and E × 53).

14 Phaeochromocytoma may be associated with the neuroectodermal diseases of which neurofibromatosis is the most frequent. This figure shows neuro-fibromata on the back. There are also cafe au lait patches.

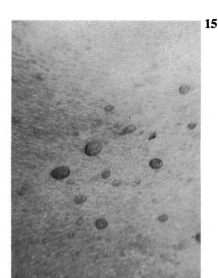

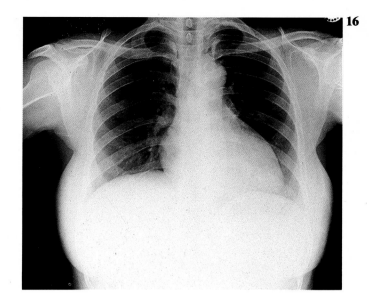

15 A magnified view of the neurofibroma on the back of the patient shown in **14**, page 42. Phaeochromocytoma may be associated with multiple endocrine adenomatas especially parathyroid and medullary carcinoma. There may be familial association.

16 Chest x-ray in patient with phaeochromocytoma. Note that the heart is enlarged with a left ventricular configuration.

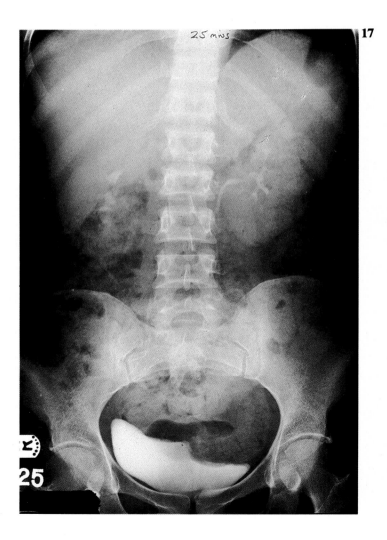

17 Intravenous urogram of a patient with right suprarenal phaeochromocytoma. Note the displacement of the right kidney with an abnormal calyceal pattern.

18 Aortogram (subtraction scan) in a patient with phaeochromocytoma. There is an abnormal vascular pattern on the right side with vessels supplying the tumour (arrowed).

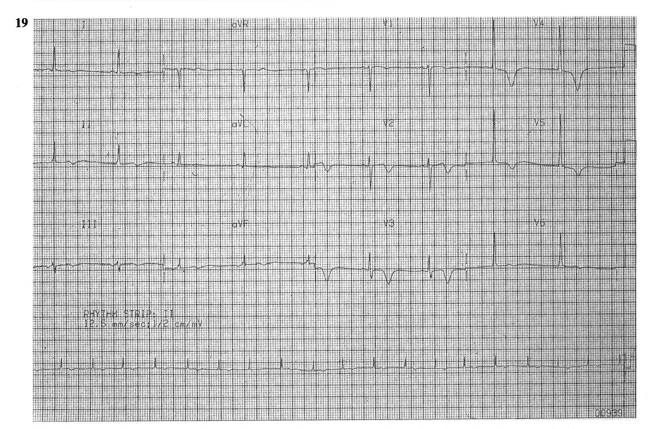

19 Electrocardiogram in patient with phaeochromocytoma. Note that there is no increased voltage of left ventricular hypertrophy, but there are widespread T wave changes suggestive of sub-endocardial ischaemia.

20 Eosinophilic adenoma of the pituitary gland from a 45-year-old woman with acromegaly. The section is stained with Biggart's eosin isamine blue showing eosinophils as red, basophils as blue/purple and chromophobes as pale grey or unstained (× 133).

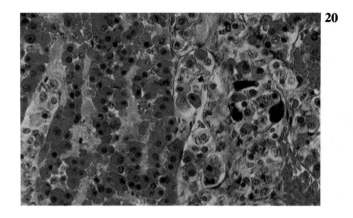

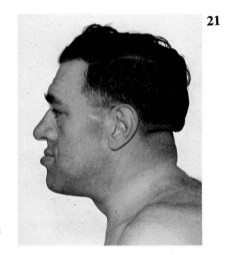

21 Acromegaly. This patient shows the typical features of acromegaly which includes thickening of the soft tissues and skin, broadening of the nose and increased prominence of the supraorbital ridges, prognathism and separation of the teeth.

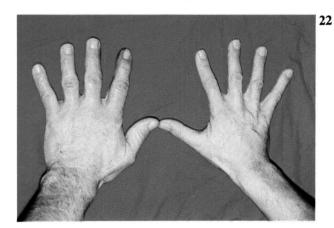

22 Acromegaly. The hands in acromegaly become larger with thickening of the soft tissues. There may be a progressive increase in ring size.

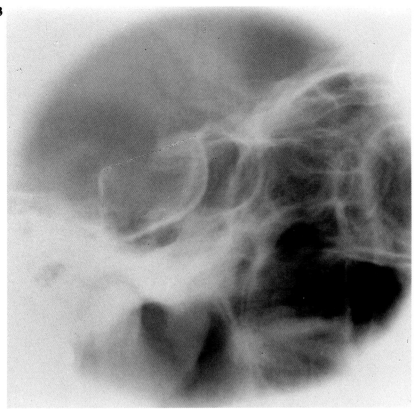

23 Coned lateral skull radiograph in a patient with acromegaly with enlargement of the pituitary fossa and a double floor.

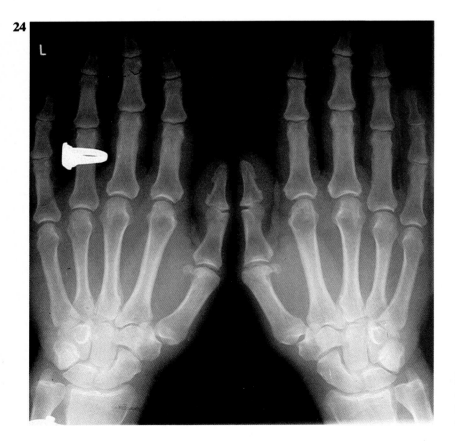

24 Hand radiograph in acromegaly. There is tufting of the terminal phalanx and thickening of the soft tissue.

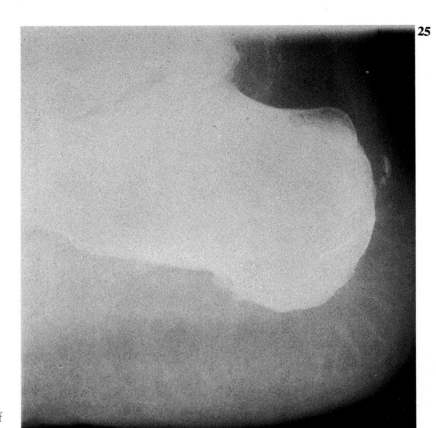

25 X-ray of the heel pad in acromegaly showing thickening of the soft tissues.

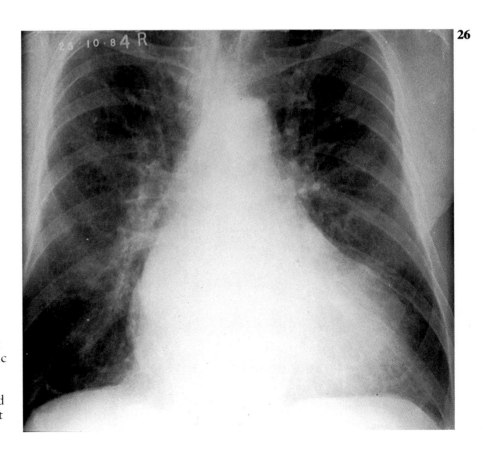

26 Chest radiograph in patient with acromegaly. There is cardiac enlargement and pulmonary venous congestion. The combination of hypertension and diabetes frequently leads to heart failure.

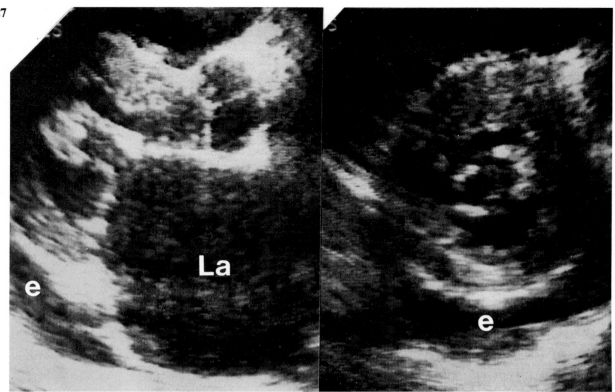

27 Two dimensional echocardiogram in patient with acromegaly. This shows a dilated and hypertrophied left ventricle with a pericardial effusion. LA – left atrium, e – effusion.

VASCULAR CAUSES OF HYPERTENSION

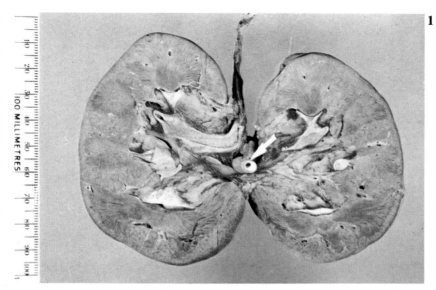

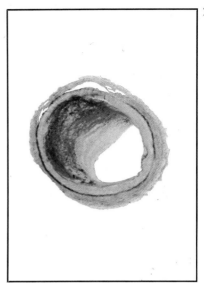

1 Atherosclerotic narrowing of the renal arteries. The arrow illustrates the deposition of lipids and cholesterol in the arterial lining producing significant narrowing of the renal artery. Note the cortex is narrowed as a result of renal ischaemia.

2 Atherosclerosis of the renal artery showing an eccentric intimal plaque containing lipid (oil red O haematoxylin × 11).

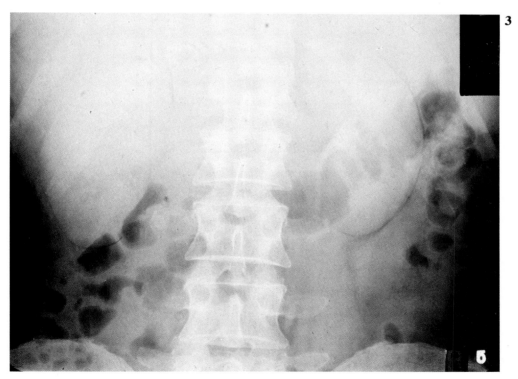

3 Five-minute intravenous urogram in renal artery stenosis showing a normal left nephrogram while the right is not visible on this early film.

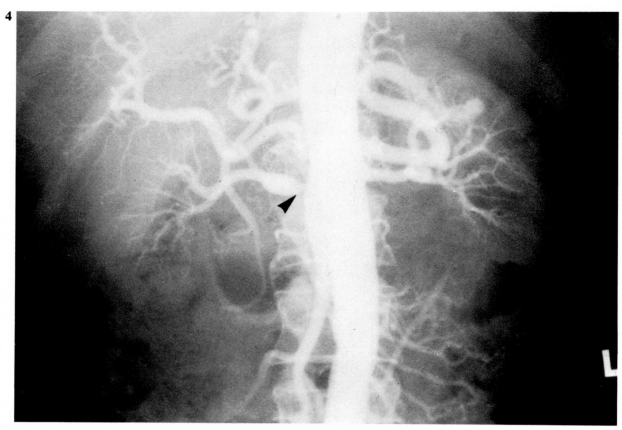

4 Descending aortogram in a patient with right renal artery stenosis (arrow).

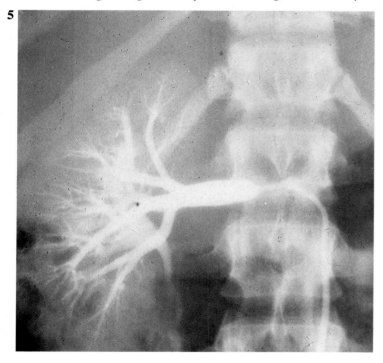

5 Selective renal arteriogram in the patient of previous figure. Note ostial stenosis of the renal artery.

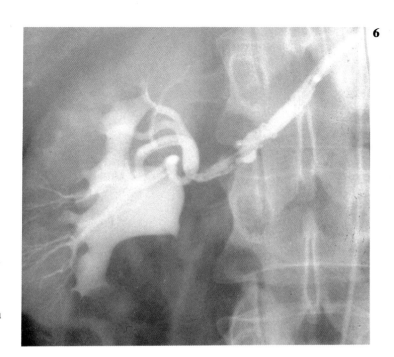

6 Selective renal arteriogram in a patient with severe fibromuscular renal artery stenosis.

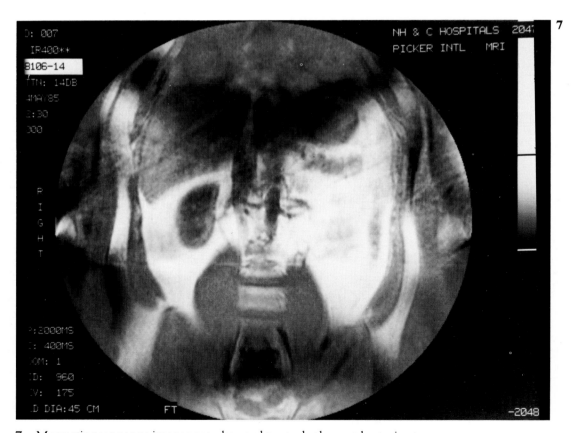

7 Magnetic resonance images may be used to study the renal arteries.

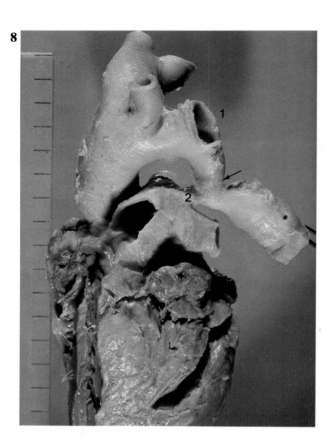

8 Gross specimen of coarctation of the aorta. The coarctation of the aorta (arrow) is present between the origin of a large left sub-clavian artery (1) and the site of attachment of a closed ductus arteriosus (2). The patient died of a cerebral haemorrhage and had hypertension in the upper part of the body.

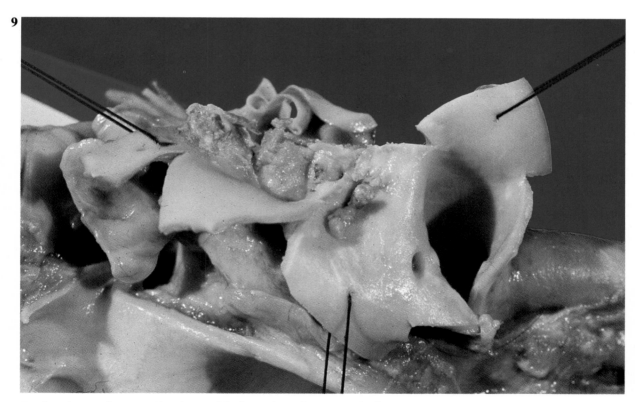

9 Specimen of coarctation in an elderly patient showing calcification and vegetations from endocarditis on the distal end of the coarctation.

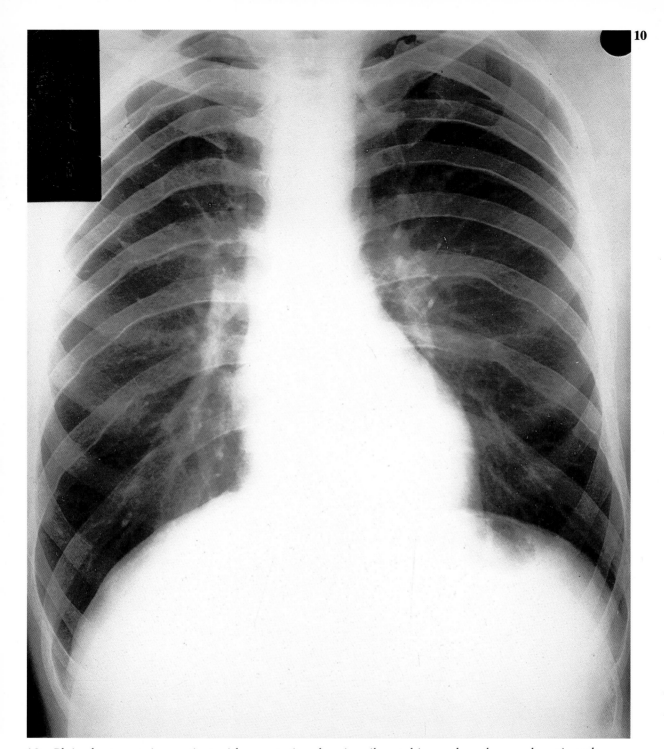

10 Plain chest x-ray in a patient with coarctation showing rib-notching and an abnormal aortic arch. Note that there is no increase in cardiac size.

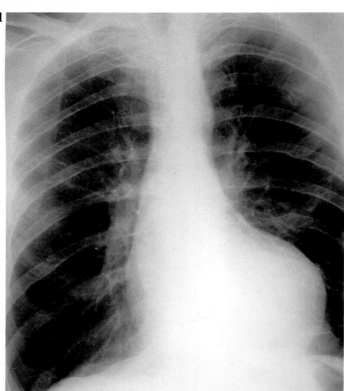

11 Cardiac enlargement due to hypertension from coarctation. There is an obvious left ventricular cardiac silhouette and absent aortic knuckle with rib-notching.

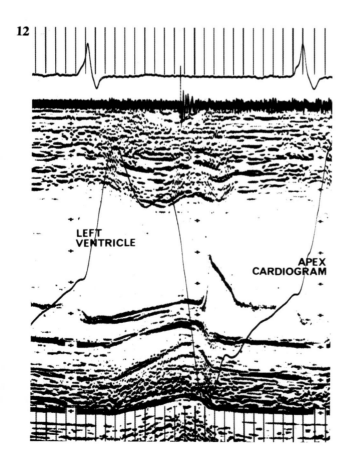

LEFT
VENTRICLE

APEX
CARDIOGRAM

12 M-Mode echocardiogram coarctation of the aorta. There is hypertrophy with a dilated poorly contracting left ventricle due to pressure overload.

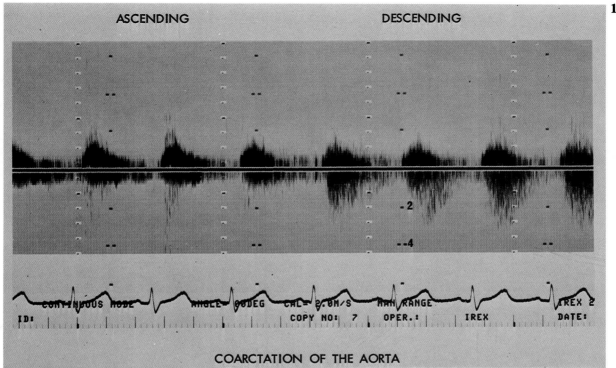

ASCENDING **DESCENDING** **13**

COARCTATION OF THE AORTA

13 Continuous wave doppler ultrasound study taken from the suprasternal notch. The blood velocity in the ascending aorta is normal (towards the transducer) and there is an increased velocity (up to 3 metres/sec, gradient 30-40 mmHg) in the descending aorta.

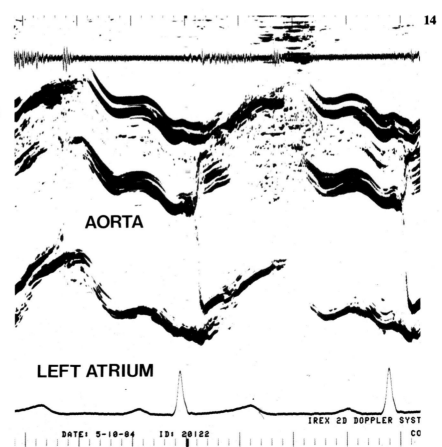

AORTA

LEFT ATRIUM

14 M-Mode echocardiogram of a bicuspid aortic valve. Note that there is an eccentric closure line of the aortic valve. This is a typical finding in patients with coarctation of the aorta and may in later life become stenotic.

55

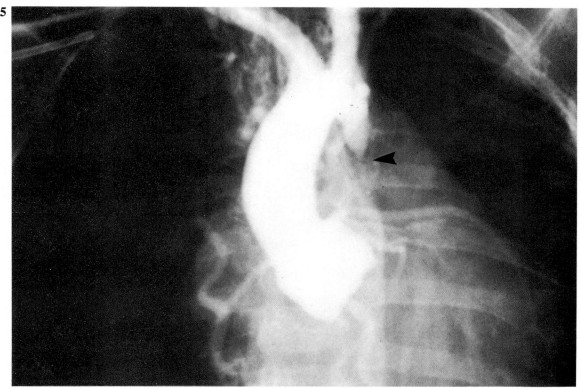

15 Aortogram (AP projection) showing an enlarged ascending aorta and a coarctation distal to the left sub-clavian (arrowed).

16 Aortogram (left anterior oblique projection) showing a coarctation (arrowed) distal to the left sub-clavian artery.

The Effects of Hypertension

The major effects of hypertension may be considered as those caused by increased blood pressure and those due to the accelerated development of atherosclerosis.

Left ventricular hypertrophy occurs as a direct consequence of increased blood pressure and would appear to be related to the severity of hypertension and its duration. Adequate anti-hypertensive therapy may lead to the reverse of the left ventricular hypertrophy. Left ventricular hypertrophy may be detected by the electro-cardiogram and chest x-ray, but these investigations are both insensitive and non-specific; echocardiography is now the method of choice. Any method employed to find left ventricular hypertrophy may constitute a major risk for the development of cardiovascular disease.

Coronary artery disease is the major cause of death in patients with hypertension and therefore should be actively sought in patients with symptoms and in those over 40 years of age. Coronary disease may be identified by the electrocardiogram at rest and on exercise, by thallium scintigraphy and by Holter monitoring. Coronary arteriography will accurately define the lesions. The major complications of coronary disease are myocardial infarction which may lead to aneurysm formation, mitral regurgitation, left venticular thrombus, heart failure and ventricular septal defect.

The clinical syndrome of heart failure may occur as a consequence of hypertension alone, but usually in combination with coronary artery disease. The left ventricular cavity is often dilated and poorly contracting, but in hypertension it may be small and hypertrophied with abnormal diastolic properties.

Peripheral vascular disease occurs in patients with hypertension and predominantly involves the aorta and leg vessels. This may be demonstrated by ultrasound and angiography.

Hypertension frequently causes dilatation of the aortic root and less commonly aortic dissection. Although aortic dissection is a rare complication of hypertension, it causes a high mortality. Both root dilatation and dissection may lead to aortic regurgitation.

The kidney may be directly involved by hypertension, initially as basement membrane thickening with arteriosclerosis and obliteration, latterly with severe parenchymal changes. This may be shown as loss of renal parenchyma by intravenous urography and may eventually lead to renal failure.

The effects of hypertension on the brain may be due to increased blood pressure alone causing haemorrhage or from accelerated atherosclerosis with cerebrovascular disease. Both may lead to the clinical features of stroke.

LEFT VENTRICULAR HYPERTROPHY

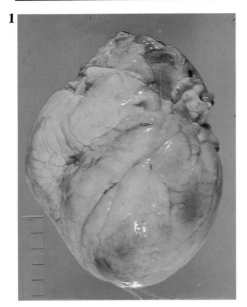

1   Anterior view of unopened
heart with considerable left
ventricular hypertrophy.

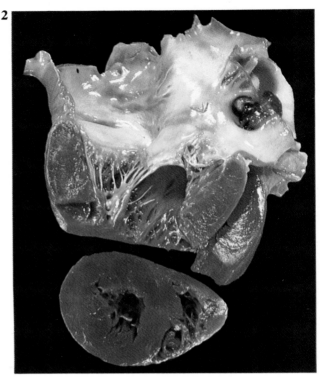

2   The heart has been displayed to demonstrate severe concentric left
ventricular hypertrophy due to longstanding systemic hypertension.

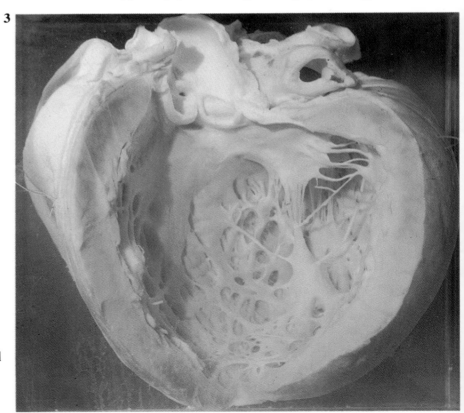

3   A dilated and hypertrophied
left ventricle from malignant
hypertension.

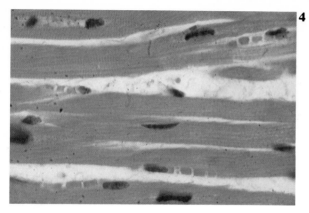

4　Histology of normal left ventricular myocardial fibres which should be compared with 5.

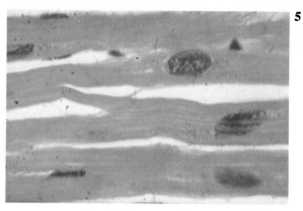

5　Hypertrophied left ventricular myocardial fibres. Note the difference in muscle fibre thickness, size and shape of nuclei (×50).

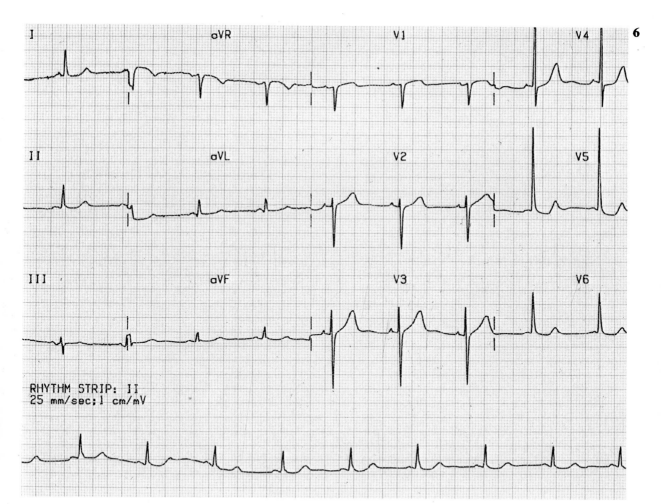

6　Electrocardiogram of borderline left ventricular hypertrophy. Note that there is increased left ventricular voltage in the precordial leads, but no ST segment changes.

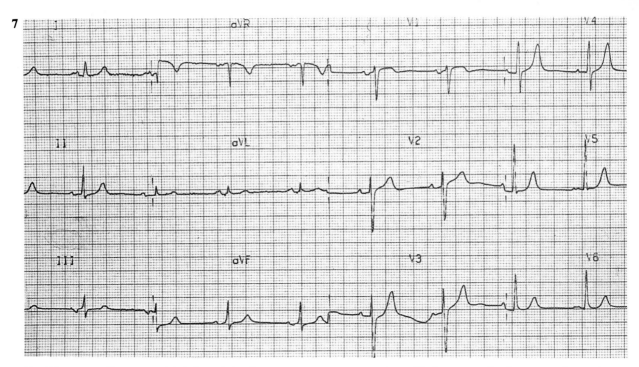

7　Electrocardiogram with left atrial enlargement as an expression of left ventricular hypertrophy without increased QRS voltage or ST segment changes. Left atrial enlargement is evidenced by biphasic P wave in lead V1.

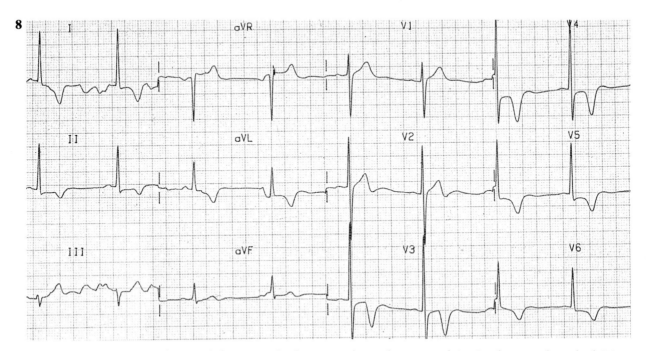

8　Electrocardiogram of severe left ventricular hypertrophy with increased QRS voltage and marked ST segment depression and T wave inversion in the left ventricular leads.

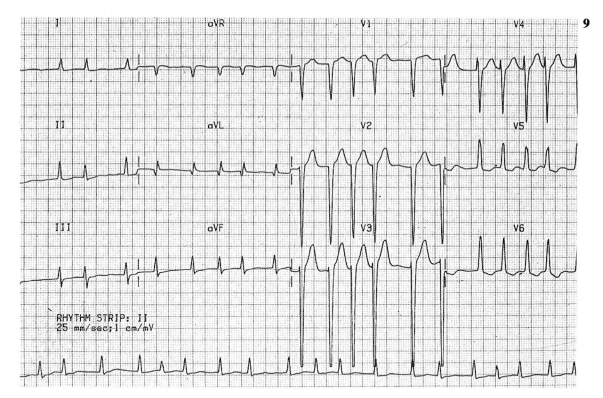

9 Electrocardiogram of severe left ventricular hypertrophy with marked ST/T wave changes, but in addition, this patient has now gone into atrial fibrillation. Atrial fibrillation is a common rhythm disorder in patients with hypertension. This patient is also on Digoxin.

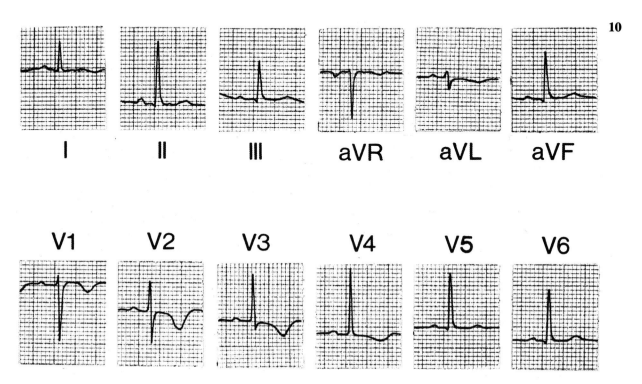

10 Occasionally the ECG may not reveal the typical features of left ventricular hypertrophy. This example is from a patient with malignant hypertension due to a phaeochromotocytoma in whom there are only T wave changes in V1–V4, but no other evidence of left ventricular hypertrophy.

11 Chest x-ray in a patient with severe hypertension. There is slight left ventricular predominance but otherwise the chest x-ray is within normal limits.

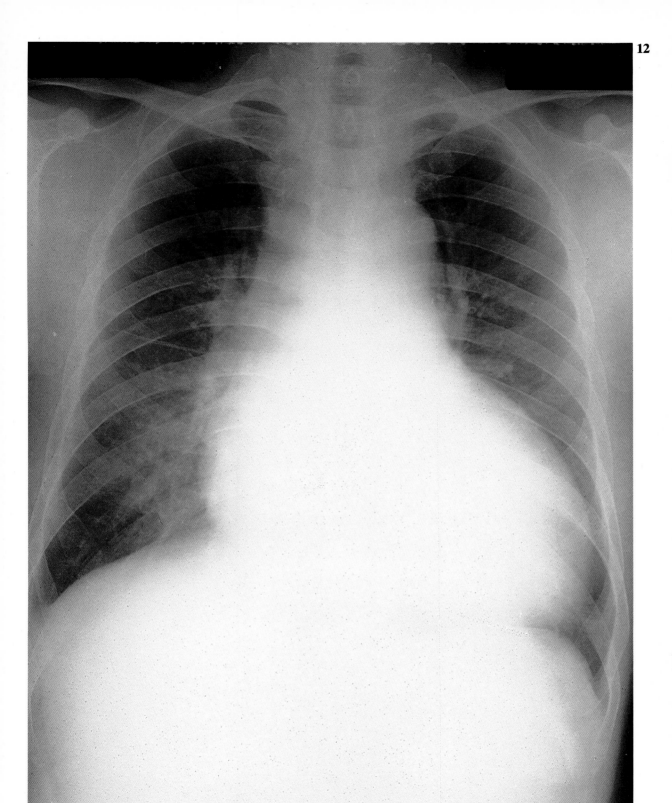

12 Chest x-ray in a patient with severe hypertension with marked left ventricular enlargement and cardiomegaly.

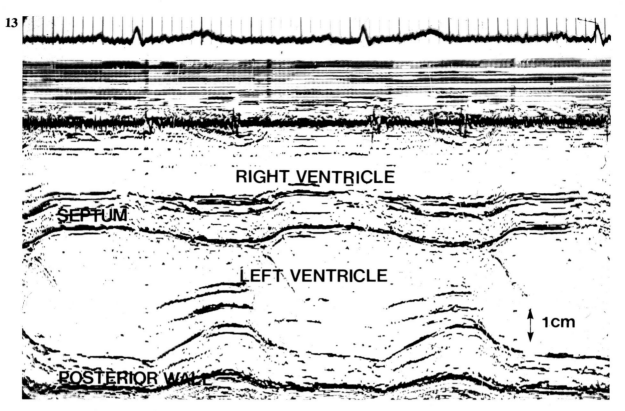

RIGHT VENTRICLE

SEPTUM

LEFT VENTRICLE

↕ 1cm

POSTERIOR WALL

13 M-Mode echocardiogram from a hypertensive patient with moderate left ventricular hypertrophy. There is increased septal and posterior left ventricular wall thickness (normal 0.7 to 1.1cm). Note that the left ventricular contraction is normal.

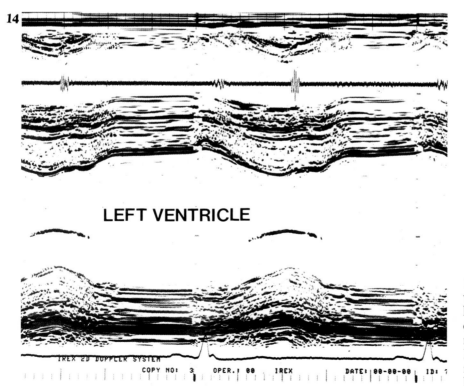

LEFT VENTRICLE

14 M-Mode echocardiogram with more severe left ventricular hypertrophy than in the previous example from a patient with moderate to severe hypertension. Left ventricular function usually remains normal with this degree of hypertrophy.

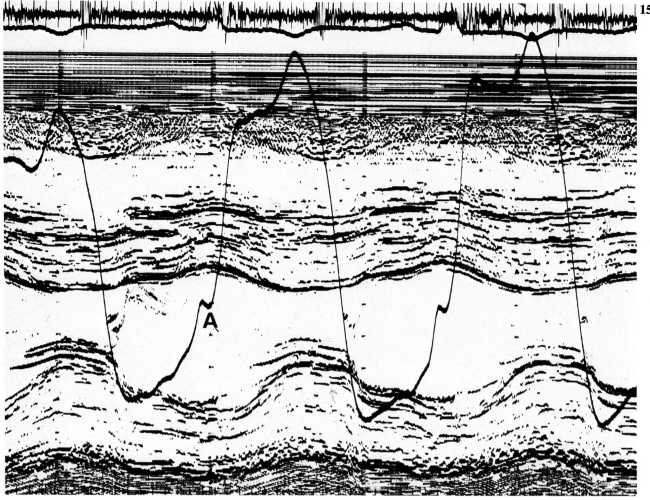

15 M-Mode echocardiogram with gross left ventricular hypertrophy; there is considerable thickening of both the septum and posterior left ventricular wall. The apex cardiogram demonstrates a tall A wave representing an increased atrial contribution to ventricular filling. The ventricular cavity is small and there is good left ventricular function.

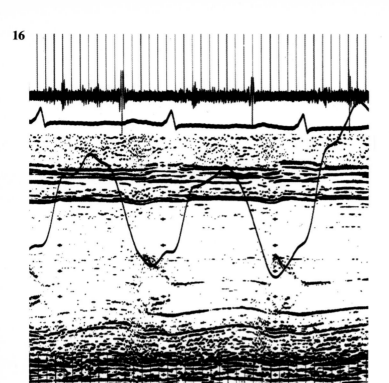

16 M-Mode echocardiogram of
a patient with severe and
longstanding hypertension who
presented with heart failure. Note
that there is thickening of the
posterior wall but the left
ventricular cavity is enlarged and
the contraction poor.

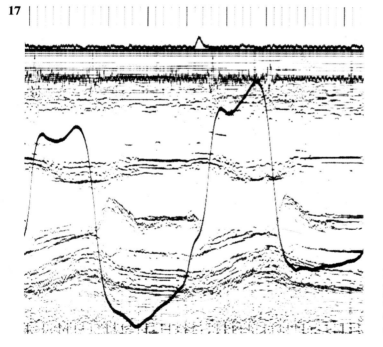

17 M-Mode echocardiogram from a
patient with malignant hypertension.
Unlike the previous examples, this patient
did not have left ventricular hypertrophy
and had normal left ventricular function.

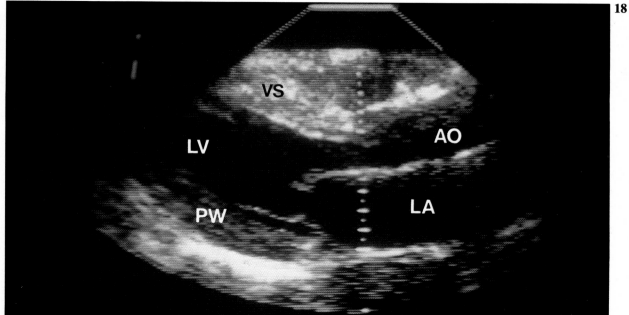

18 Two dimensional echocardiogram, parasternal long axis view, showing left ventricular hypertrophy with a small left ventricular cavity. Note that the septum is thicker than the posterior wall. Asymmetrical septal hypertrophy may be seen occasionally in hypertension. VS–ventricular septum; PW–posterior wall; LV–left ventricle; Ao–aorta; LA–left atrium.

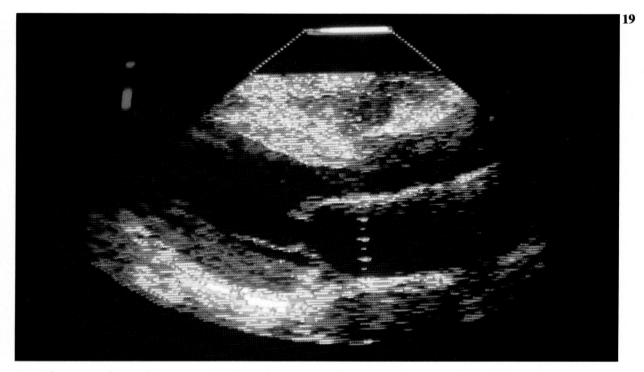

19 The same echocardiogram as **18** above, but processed using a colour encoded technique. Normal echo amplitude (cyan and green) is seen in the posterior wall but the septum has blue, red and white echoes indicative of increased myocardial collagen content (note similar to the fibrous posterior pericardium).

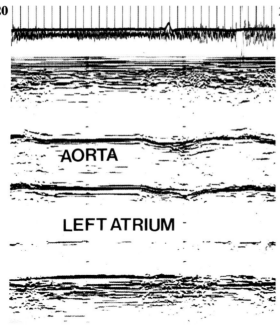

AORTA

LEFT ATRIUM

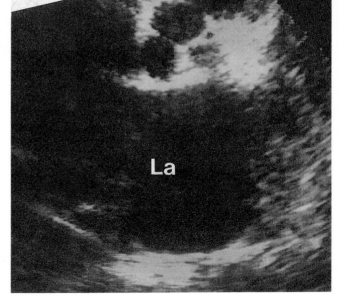

La

20 M-Mode echocardiogram of moderate left atrial enlargement in a patient with severe left ventricular hypertrophy. Aortic root motion in this particular example is rather reduced reflecting poor cardiac contraction.

21 Two dimensional echocardiogram (same patient as in 20, this page) in a short axis parasternal view. It may be noted that the aortic valve is tricuspid and the left atrium enlarged. La–left atrium.

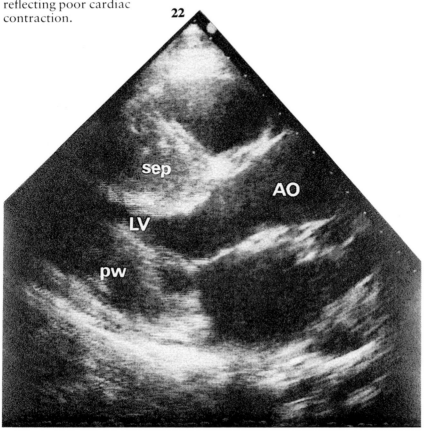

sep

AO

LV

pw

22 Two dimensional echocardiogram parasternal long axis view in a hypertensive patient with an enlarged left atrium. In addition, there is gross septal and posterior wall hypertrophy. Sep–septum; PW–posterior wall; LV–left ventricle; Ao–aorta.

23 Pressure trace recorded from a patient with hypertension and left ventricular hypertrophy. There were clinical signs of heart failure. There was a grossly elevated left ventricular end-diastolic and pulmonary capillary wedge pressures (PCWP).

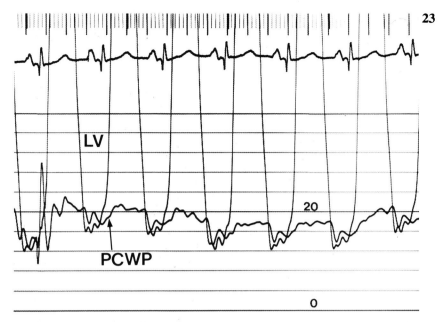

24 Left ventricular angiogram in anterior posterior position showing severe left ventricular hypertrophy in a hypertensive child.

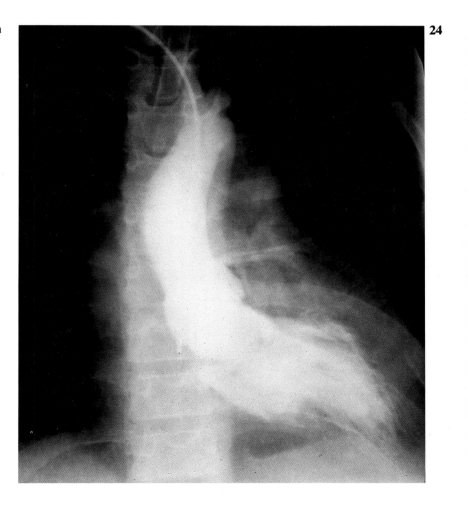

25

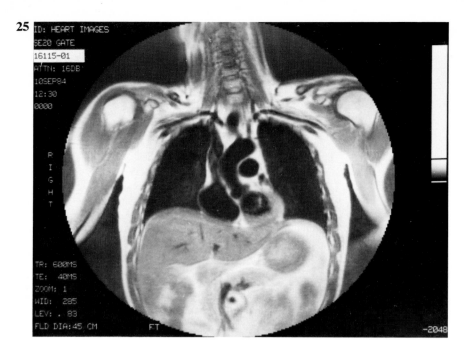

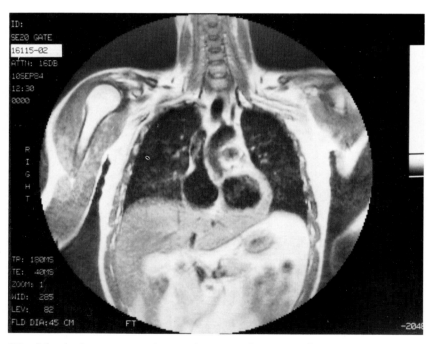

25   Magnetic resonance images in coronal section of a normal man in systole and diastole.

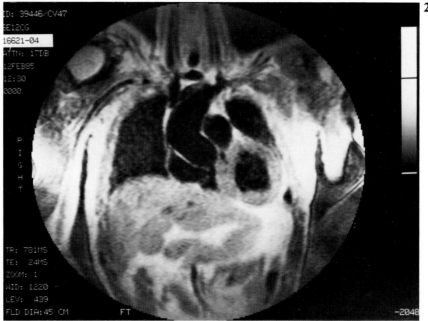

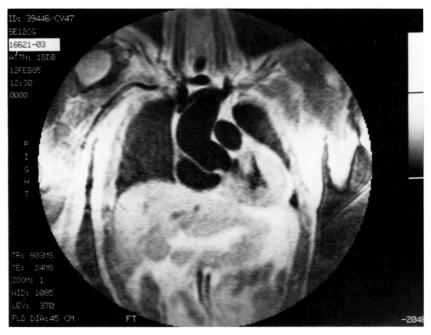

26 Magnetic resonance images in systole and diastole in a patient with left ventricular hypertrophy due to hypertension.

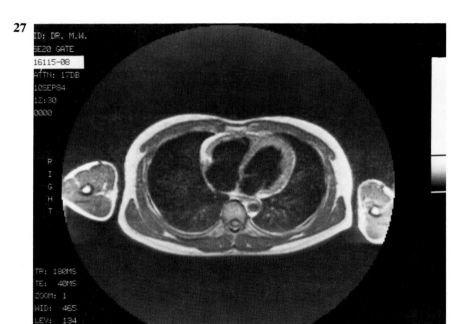

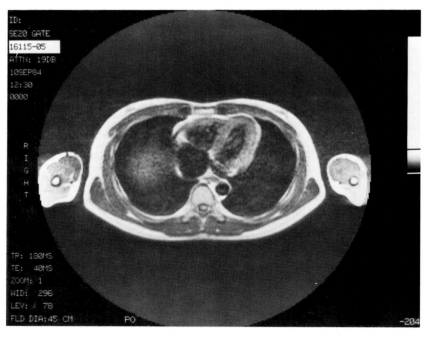

27 Magnetic resonance images in systole and diastole. Transverse
section in normal man.

28

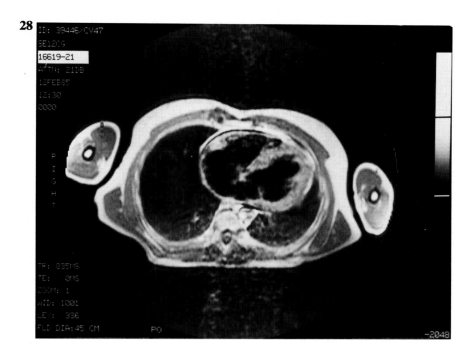

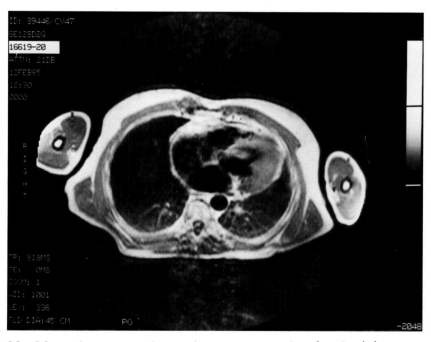

28 Magnetic resonance images in transverse section showing left ventricular hypertrophy due to hypertension.

CORONARY ARTERY DISEASE

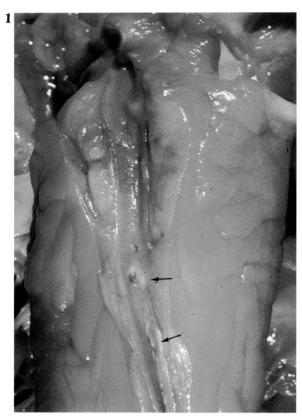

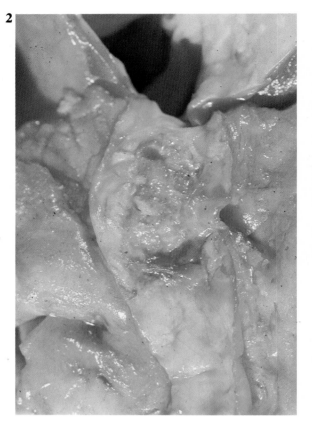

1   Coronary artery atheroma. A left anterior descending coronary artery opened longitudinally to show the distribution of early atheromatous plaques around the openings of its branches (arrows).

2   Coronary artery atheroma. A right coronary artery opened longitudinally to show an area of severe disease with atheromatous material exuding into the lumen. At the lower end of the plaque there is a haemorrhage in the wall and an adjacent intimal tear.

3   Coronary artery atheroma. Cross-section of a coronary artery severely affected by atheroma stained by haematoxylin and eosin. The lumen, markedly reduced by atheroma, was terminally occluded by thrombus but in preparation of the sections this has shrunk away from the intima. The histological features that may be present in varying proportion in any severely diseased artery, associated with destruction of the normal architecture of the wall are lipid and foam cells, fibrin, cholesterol crystals, chronic inflammatory cell infiltrate, increased vascularisation, haemorrhage, thrombosis, fibrosis, necrosis and calcification.

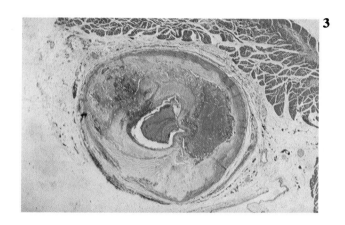

3

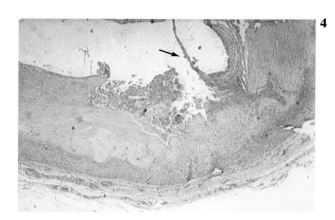

4

4   Coronary artery atheroma. Close-up of an intimal rupture (arrow) in a coronary artery with severe atheroma. This type of tear, usually overlying an area of 'soft' atheromatous tissue may be an important initiating factor in thrombosis.

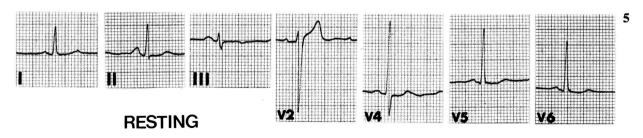

5

RESTING

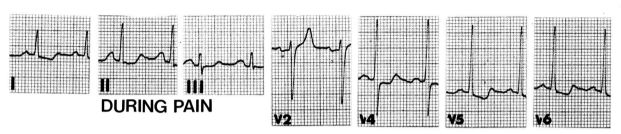

DURING PAIN

5   Electrocardiogram. During anginal pain there are usually ST and T wave changes recorded on the ECG. Above is the normal resting electrocardiogram but during pain (below) ST and T wave changes can be seen, particularly involving the lateral chest leads.

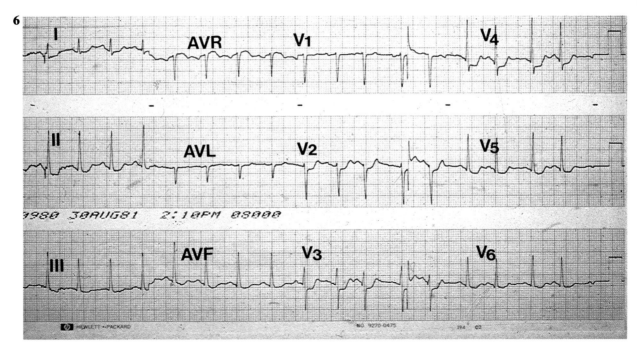

6 Exercise electrocardiogram. At rest the ECG may be normal but on exercise, due to the development of myocardial ischaemia, there are ST segment changes. Here ST segment changes are widespread.

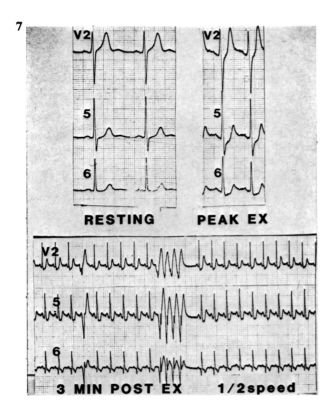

7 Electrocardiogram. Very occasionally, with the induction of ST segment changes, and myocardial ischaemia, ventricular arrhythmias may occur. They may occur during exercise or even after exercise has been discontinued, as in this example when they were recorded 3 minutes after the end of exercise.

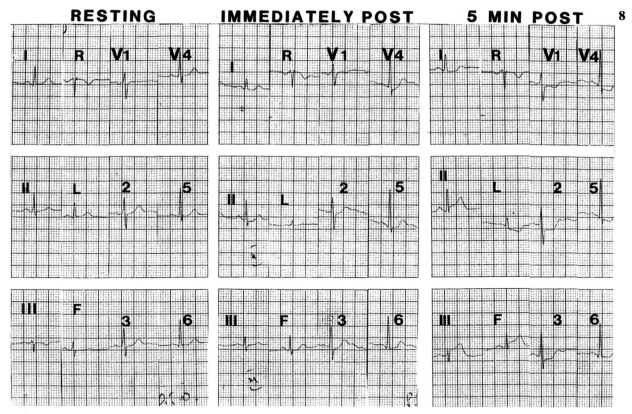

8   Electrocardiogram. Although ST segment depression is the most common finding, occasionally ST segment elevation may be recorded, either during exercise or on recovery. The development of ST segment elevation as opposed to ST segment depression usually indicates very severe proximal disease of at least one of the major coronary arteries.

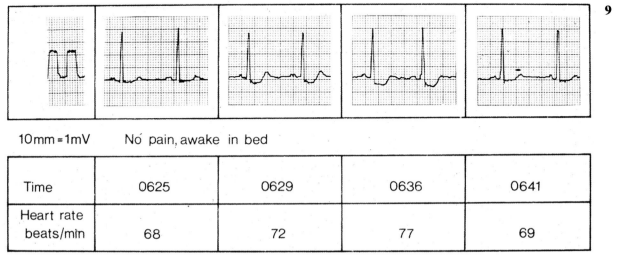

10mm = 1mV   No pain, awake in bed

Time	0625	0629	0636	0641
Heart rate beats/min	68	72	77	69

9   Ambulatory monitoring. ST segment changes can also be recorded using ambulatory monitoring. This example shows the development of ST segment depression during angina in a patient with severe coronary artery disease.

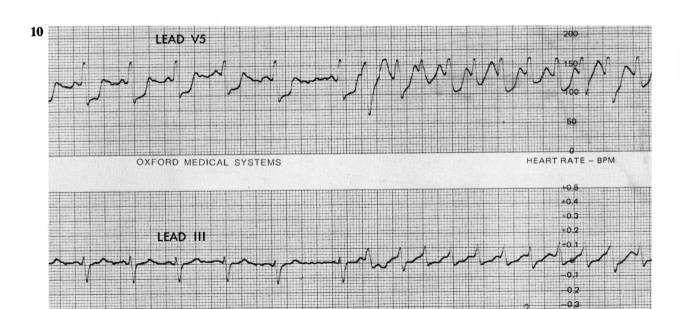

LEAD V5

OXFORD MEDICAL SYSTEMS

HEART RATE – BPM

200
150
100
50
0

+0.5
+0.4
+0.3
+0.2
+0.1
0
-0.1
-0.2
-0.3
-0.4

LEAD III

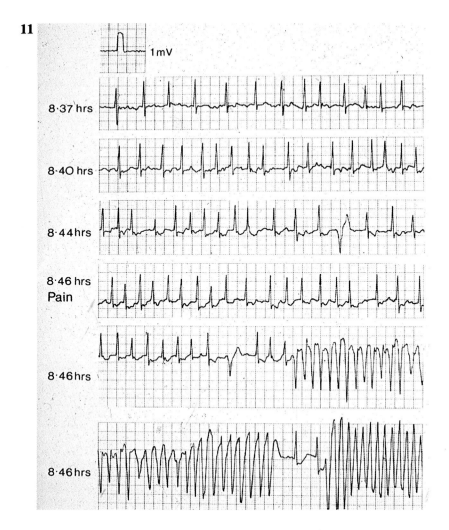

1mV

8.37 hrs

8.40 hrs

8.44 hrs

8.46 hrs
Pain

8.46 hrs

8.46 hrs

10 Ambulatory monitoring. Occasionally during episodes of myocardial ischaemia and ST segment depression, ventricular arrhythmias may occur. In this example the patient developed angina and ST segment depression before the onset of ventricular tachycardia.

11 Ambulatory monitoring. During myocardial ischaemia sudden death may occur and this is usually due to the development of ventricular fibrillation.

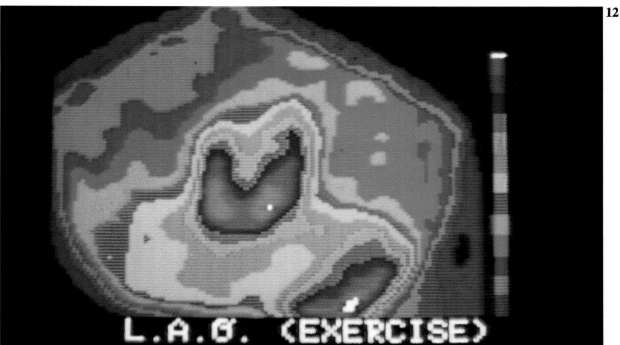

L.A.0. (EXERCISE)

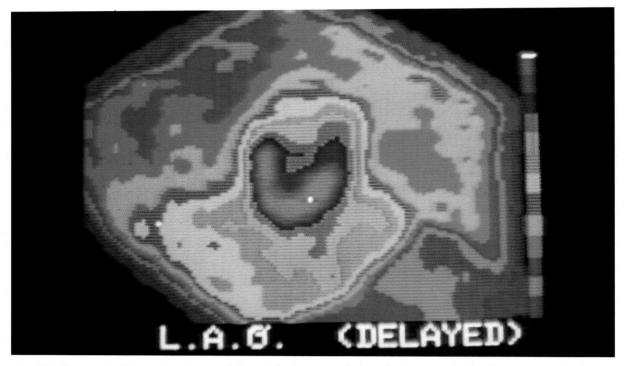

L.A.0. (DELAYED)

12 Thallium scintillography. Areas of diminished myocardial perfusion can also be demonstrated using Thallium 201 scintillography. This figure shows a normal thallium scan recorded during (top) and after (bottom) exercise in the left anterior oblique position (LAO). There is an even distribution of perfusion to the myocardium.

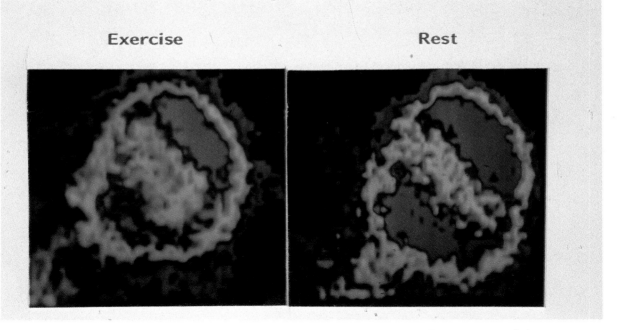

13 Thallium scintillography. On exercise in patients with coronary artery disease, areas of absent perfusion will be seen using thallium scintillography. This is shown in the left hand panel where there is an apical defect. At rest on reperfusion four and a half hours later, the defect is no longer present.

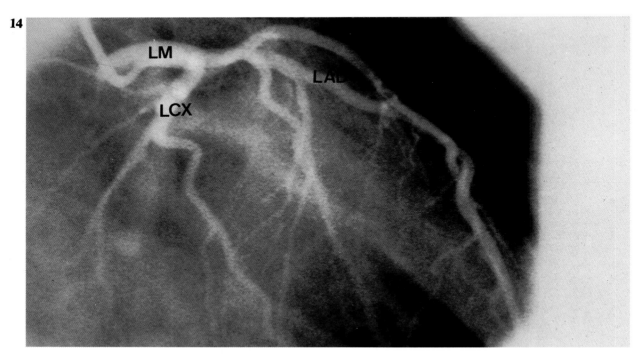

14 The coronary artery anatomy can in life be best demonstrated using coronary arteriography. This is a normal left coronary arteriogram in the right anterior oblique projection. LM–left main stem; LCX–left circumflex; LAD–left anterior descending.

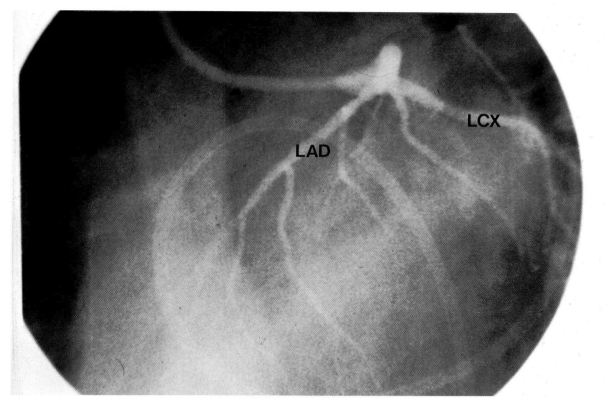

15 A normal left coronary artery in the left anterior oblique projection. LCX–left circumflex; LAD–left anterior descending.

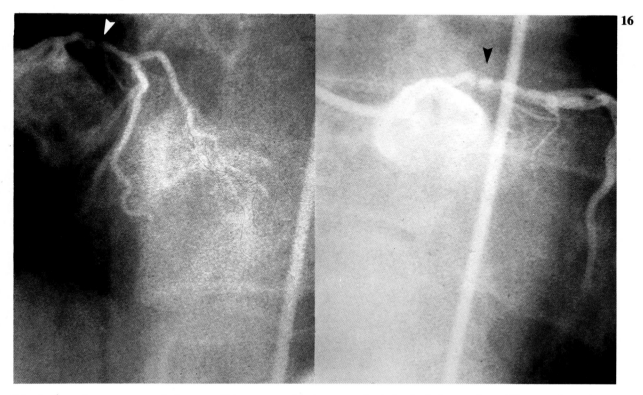

16 Left main stem stenosis (arrowed) in two projections: on the left, the left anterior oblique and on the right, the antero-posterior projection.

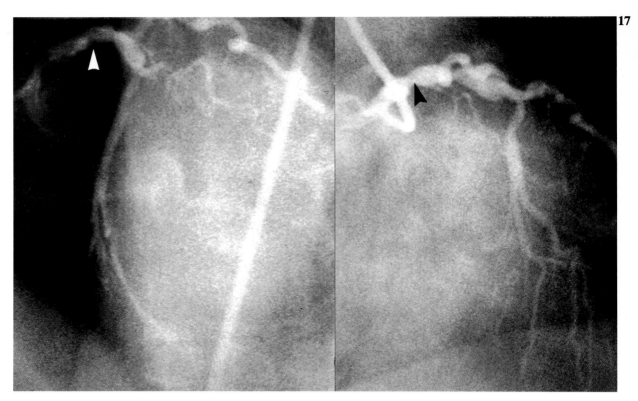

17   A tight left main stem stenosis (arrowed) in two projections.

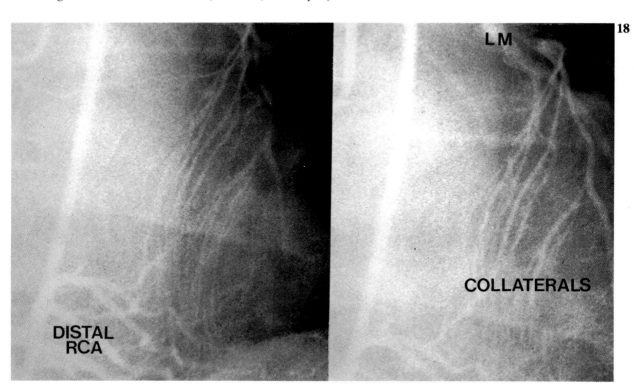

18   Blocked left main stem stenosis which is demonstrated by injection of the right coronary artery (RCA) and the whole of the left coronary artery filling by collateral circulation. Both views are in the right anterior oblique projection. The left hand panel shows the early phase in which the collaterals can be clearly seen and the right hand panel shows contrast already in the left main (LM) coronary artery.

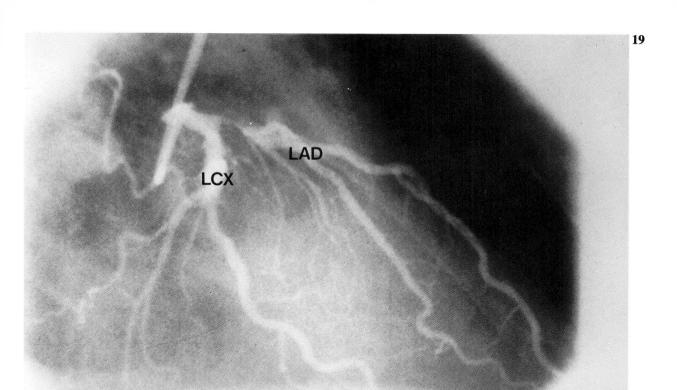

19 Left anterior descending (LAD) coronary artery stenosis seen in the right anterior oblique projection. LCX–left circumflex.

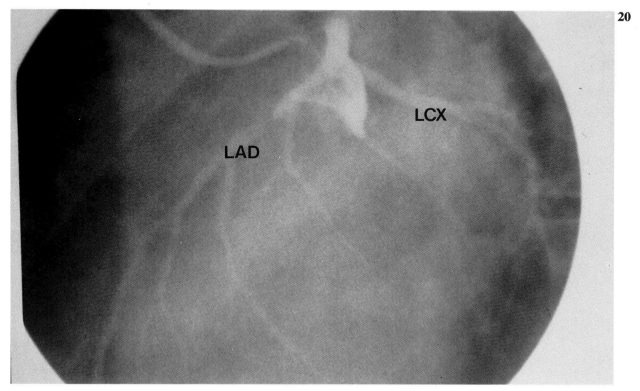

20 Left anterior descending (LAD) stenosis in the left anterior oblique projection. LCX–left circumflex.

83

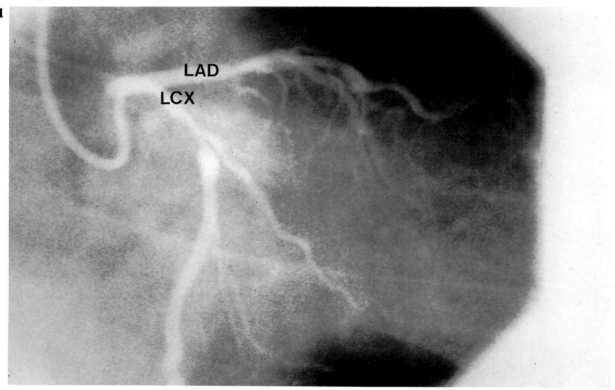

21 Circumflex lesion in the left anterior oblique projection. LCX–left circumflex; LAD–left anterior descending.

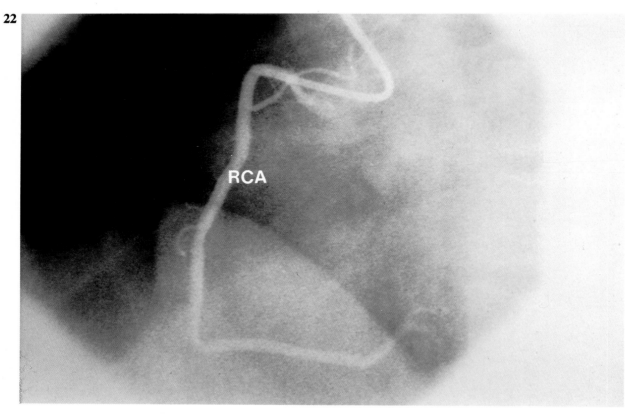

22 A normal right coronary artery (RCA) in the left anterior oblique projection.

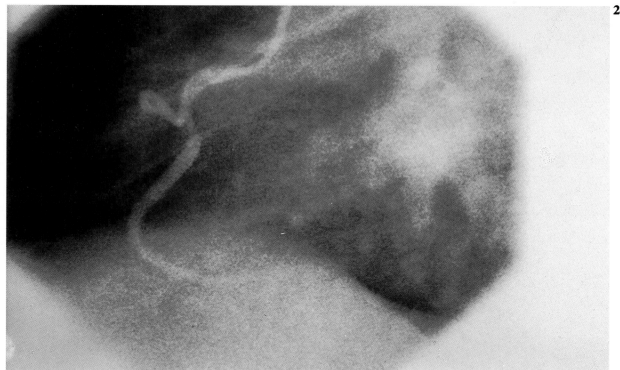

23   An isolated right coronary artery stenosis in the left anterior oblique projection.

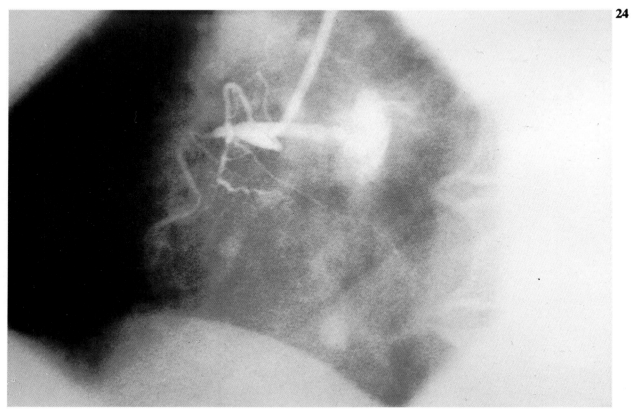

24   A blocked right coronary artery in the left anterior oblique projection.

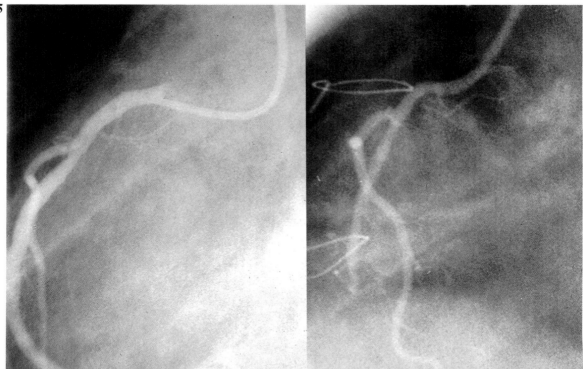

25 Progression of coronary artery atheroma. On the left hand panel a normal right coronary artery is seen. In the right hand panel taken three years later, atheroma has developed so that the right coronary artery is now blocked two thirds of the way down its course.

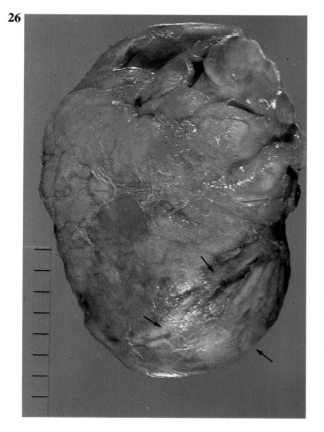

26 Pathology of myocardial infarction. An apical and anterior wall myocardial infarct (arrow) which resulted from occlusion of the left anterior descending coronary artery. In addition there is generalised fibrinous pericarditis.

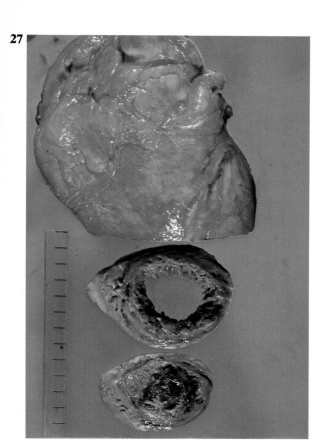

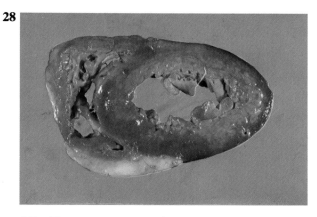

27 Transverse ventricular slices cut from the apex of the heart illustrated in the previous figure. The infarct involves the whole of the apical slice but in the upper slice the infarction is confined to the anterior wall of the left ventricle and the anterior half of the inter-ventricular septum. Note also the endocardial thrombus.

28 Pallor is the initial gross change that can be seen in the area of infarction and is usually apparent about 12-15 hours after the onset of ischaemia. This transverse ventricular slice shows extensive areas of pallor in the left ventricular wall following occlusion of the main trunk of the left coronary artery in a heart with a left dominant pattern.

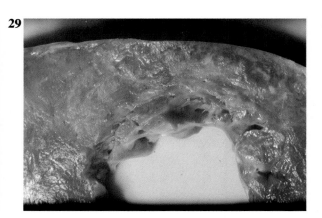

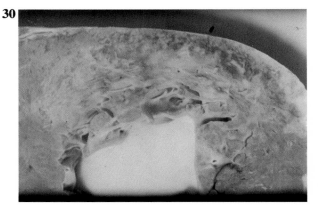

29 By about 36 hours, the area of pallor becomes surrounded by a haemorrhagic zone as in the posterior wall of the left ventricle of this heart.

30 The haemorrhagic zone of the infarct illustrated in the previous figure (29) is more clearly seen after photographing the specimen under water.

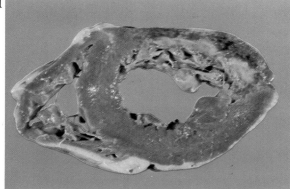

31 The centre of the infarct becomes more opaque and the haemorrhagic border more distinct after approximately 3 - 4 days.

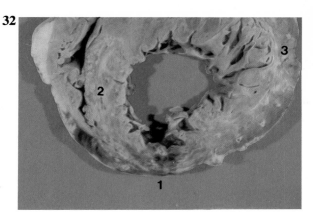

32 An area of ischaemic myocardium may enlarge, possibly due to extension of coronary thrombosis, some time after the initial infarction. In this transverse ventricular slice the infarcted area has extended from the initially damaged anterior wall (1) into the anterior half of the inter-ventricular septum (2). Sub-endocardial fibrosis (3) and thinning of the lateral wall indicates a previous area of myocardial ischaemia.

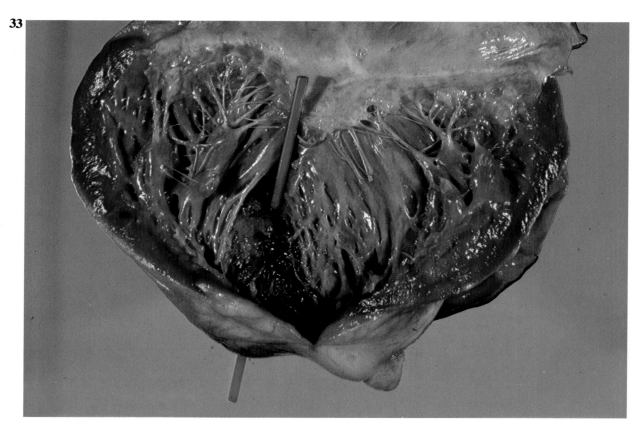

33 Mural thrombus. A left ventricle opened to show a recently formed mural thrombus attached to an area of infarction in the anterior apical region. Rupture of the wall has also occurred.

Ventricular aneurysm. Aneurysms may
~elop following thinning and weakness of the
arcted myocardial wall. This figure illustrates a
y large apical aneurysm of the left ventricle
d with a laminated thrombus. The patient had
story of a myocardial infarction 4 years
viously.

34

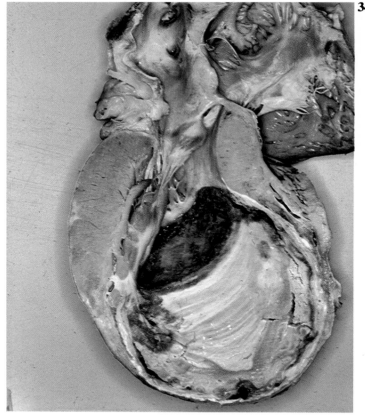

35

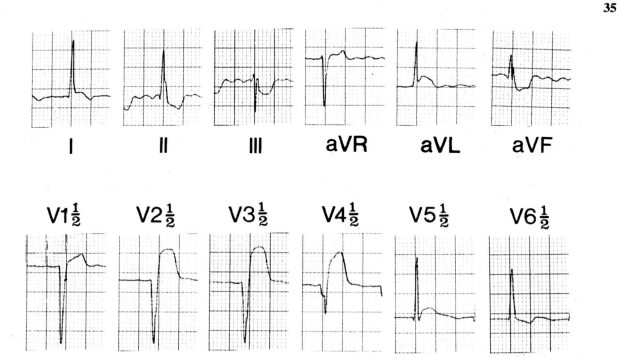

35 Electrocardiogram from a patient with an antero-lateral myocardial infarction. Q waves are present
from V1-V4 with ST segment elevation in the anterior leads and also in the lateral limb leads. There is
reciprocal ST segment depression to be seen in the inferior leads.

89

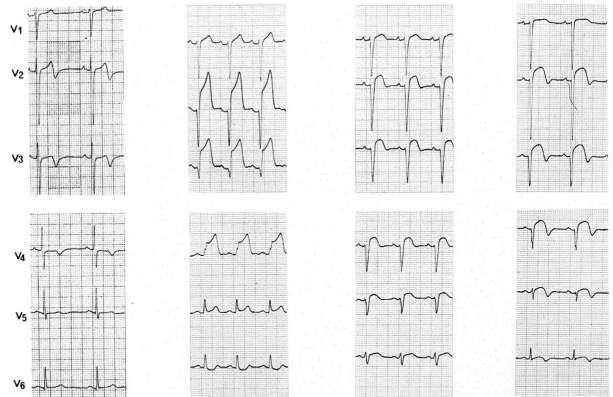

V1

V2

V3

V4

V5

V6

36 Electrocardiogram showing the evolution of an anterior myocardial infarction. On the left is the resting ECG before the patient presented with acute chest pain showing evidence of a probable previous subendocardial infarction. There is subsequently the development of ST segment elevation, then Q waves develop and finally there are Q waves with ST segment elevation and T wave inversion.

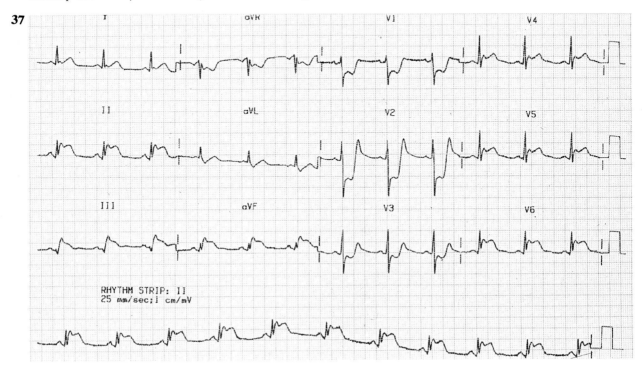

I aVR V1 V4

II aVL V2 V5

III aVF V3 V6

RHYTHM STRIP: II
25 mm/sec; 1 cm/mV

37 Electrocardiogram in inferior myocardial infarction seen in the early stages with marked ST segment elevation in the inferior leads and also in the lateral chest leads. Reciprocal ST segment depression in the anterior chest leads is also present. At this stage Q waves have not yet developed.

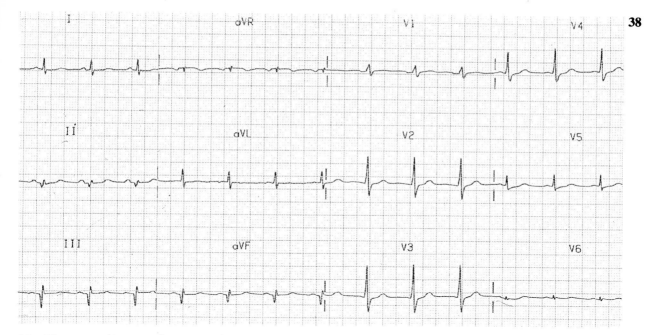

38 Electrocardiogram showing inferior myocardial infarction at a later stage than in **37**, page 90 with the development of Q waves; the ST segments have now reverted to normal.

39 Electrocardiogram showing a subendocardial anterior myocardial infarction; there is gross T wave inversion in the anterior chest leads but there are no Q waves.

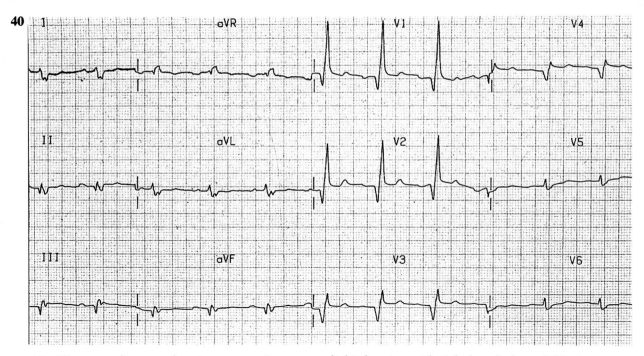

40 Electrocardiogram showing an anterior myocardial infarction with right bundle branch block.

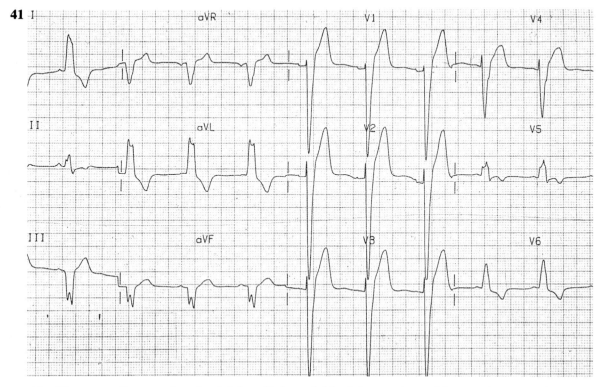

41 Electrocardiogram showing left bundle branch block in a patient with a previous anterior myocardial infarction. Evidence of the previous infarction is obscured by the left bundle branch block.

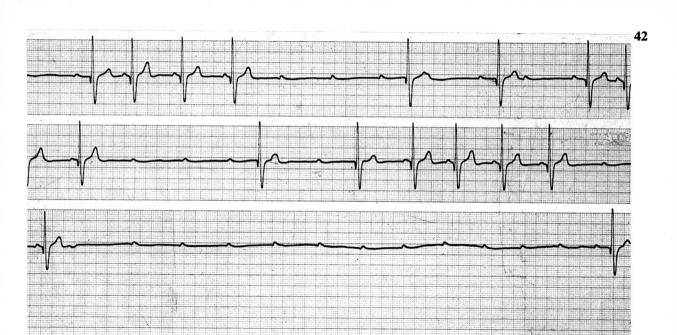

42

42 Electrocardiogram. This is an important complication of acute myocardial infarction in which there is complete heart block leading to asystole (shown in monitor leads).

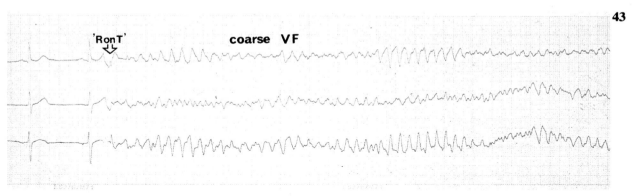

43

43 Electrocardiogram. Another important complication, ie an R on T ventricular ectopic followed by ventricular fibrillation.

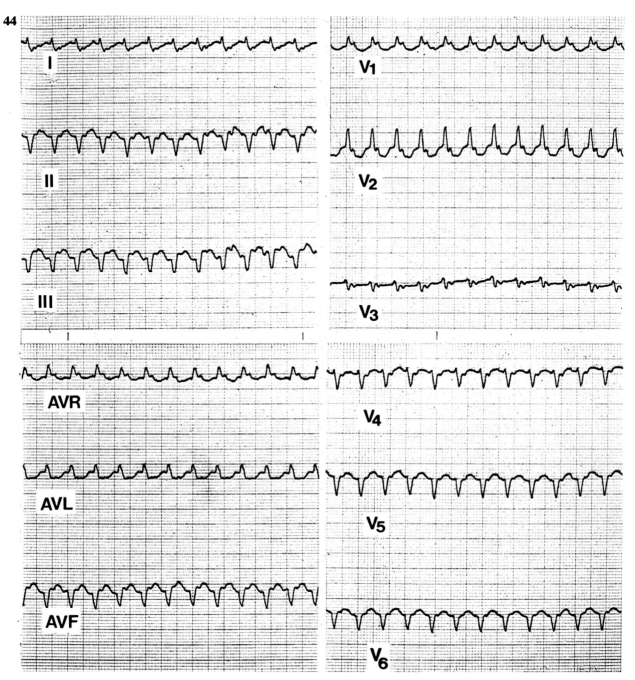

44 Electrocardiogram showing inferior myocardial infarction in a patient with the development of supra-ventricular tachycardia.

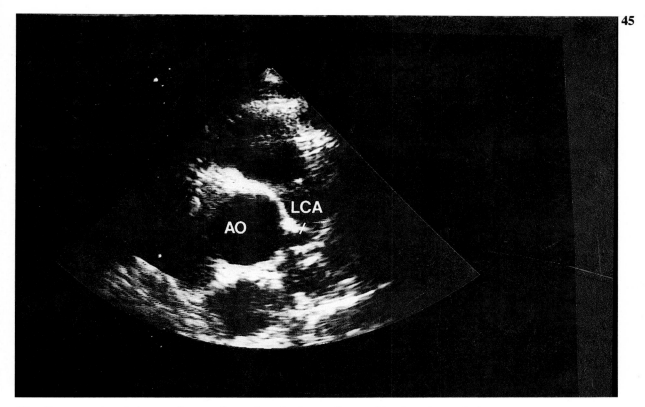

45 Cross-sectional short axis two dimensional echocardiographic view through the aortic root (AO) showing the aorta in cross-section and the left coronary artery (LCA). Echocardiography may be used to study only the proximal portion of the left coronary artery.

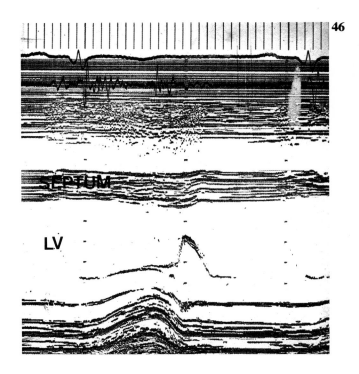

46 M-Mode echocardiogram showing a moderately enlarged left ventricular (LV) cavity with impaired left ventricular function and poor septal motion (flat septum due to previous septal infarction).

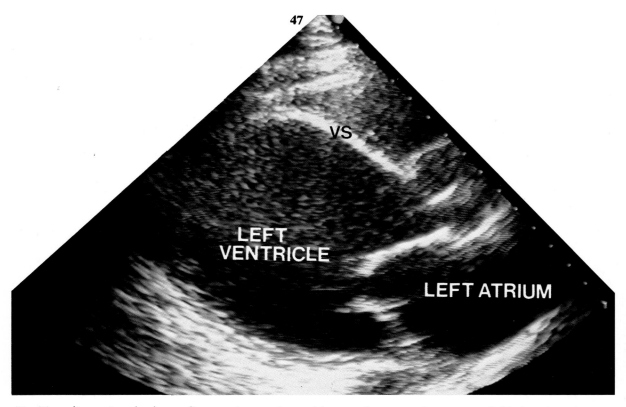

47 Two dimensional echocardiogram in a patient with a previous anterior myocardial infarction, the septum (VS) is thin and the left ventricular cavity dilated.

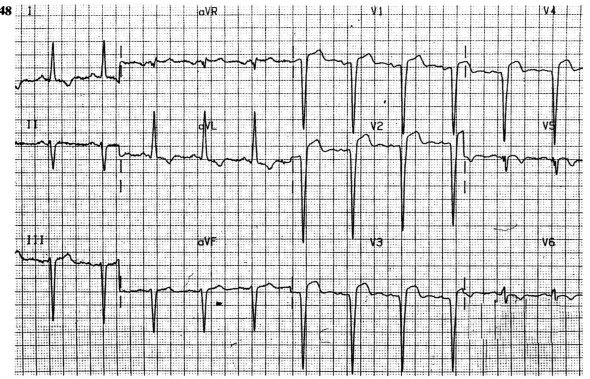

48 Electrocardiogram in a patient with a previous anterior myocardial infarction who developed a left ventricular aneurysm. There are Q waves and persistent ST segment elevation in the anterior chest leads.

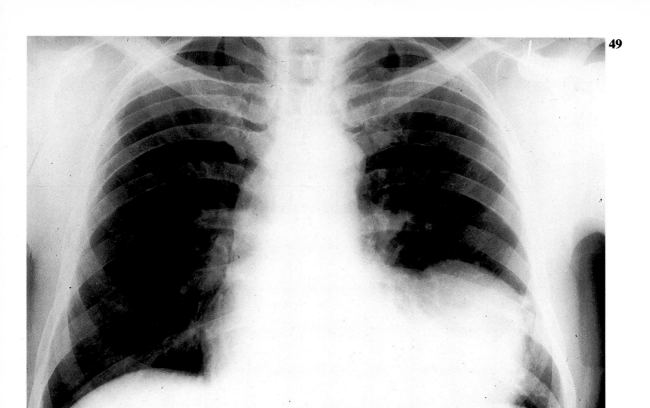

49 Chest x-ray showing a huge
left ventricular aneurysm which
can be seen as a bulge on the left
ventricular free wall.

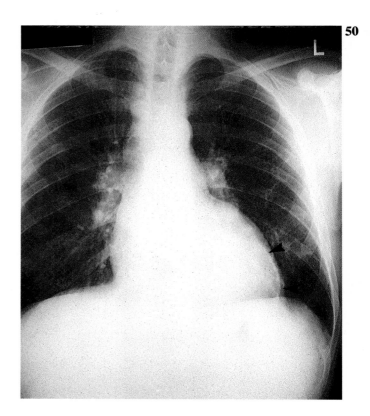

50 Chest x-ray showing a
smaller left ventricular aneurysm
than in the previous example but
there is linear calcification of the
aneurysm (arrowed).

51

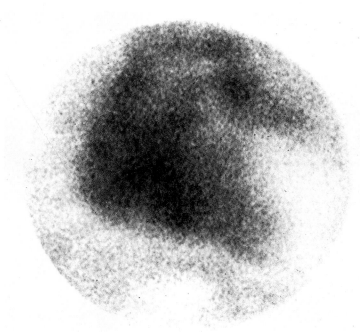

51 Technetium 99M labelled gated blood pool scan showing the left ventricle with a large left ventricular aneurysm.

52

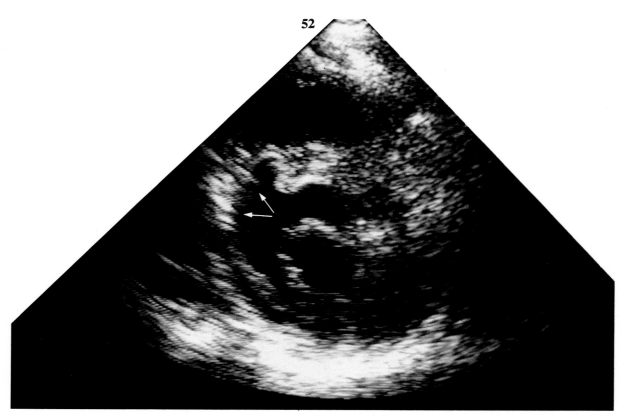

52 Two dimensional echocardiographic short axis view through the left ventricle showing a septal aneurysm (arrowed).

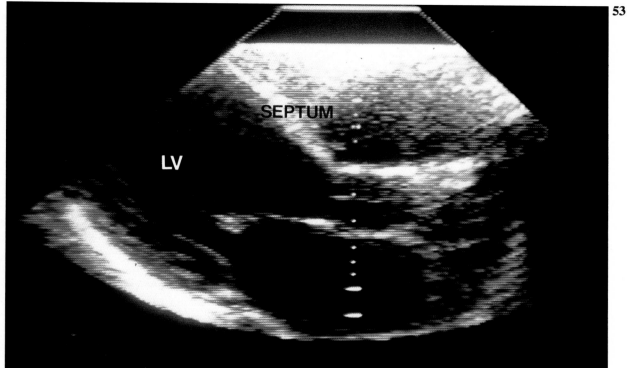

53 Two dimensional echocardiographic long axis view showing an aneurysm of the septum, shown as a thin (and immobile) structure. LV–left ventricle.

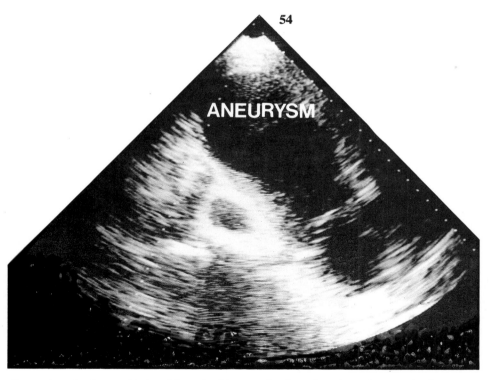

54 Two dimensional echocardiographic apical long axis view showing a huge apical aneurysm.

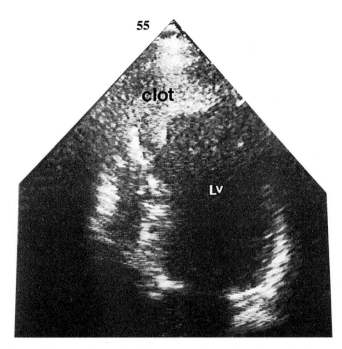

55 Two dimensional echocardiographic apical long axis view showing apical aneurysm with left ventricular clot.

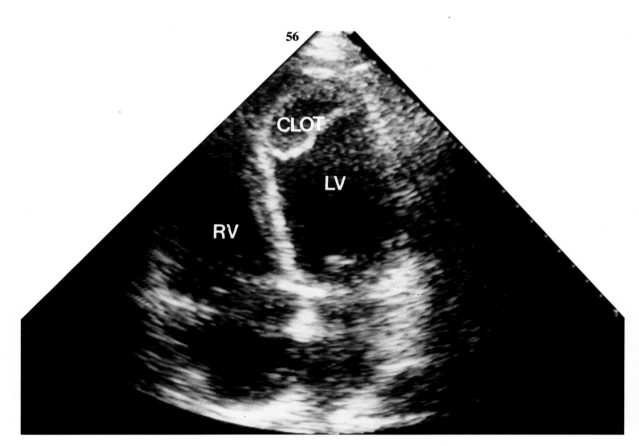

56 Two dimensional echocardiographic four chamber view showing a mobile, liquefying clot at the apex of the left ventricle. LV–left ventricle; RV–right ventricle.

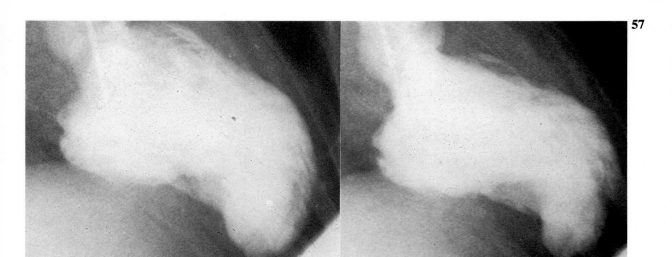

57   Ventricular angiogram showing an apical left ventricular aneurysm with a systolic frame (right) and a diastolic frame (left).

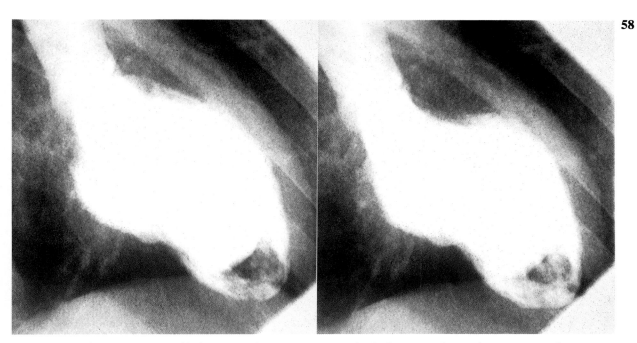

58   Ventricular angiogram of left ventricular aneurysm in which there is a clot in the aneurysmal sac. On the left is a diastolic frame and on the right is a systolic frame.

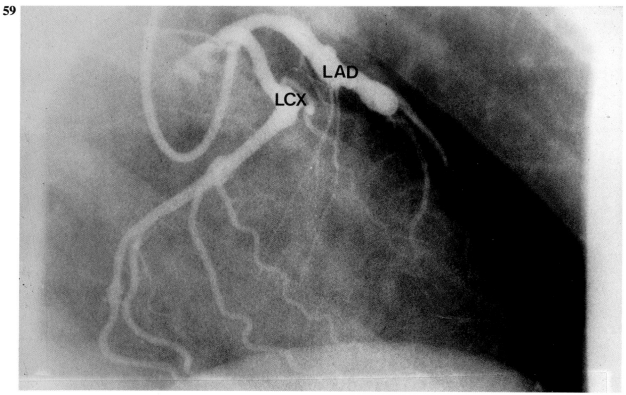

59 Coronary arteriogram in a patient with an antero-apical left ventricular aneurysm in which the left anterior descending (LAD) coronary artery is blocked. LCX–left circumflex.

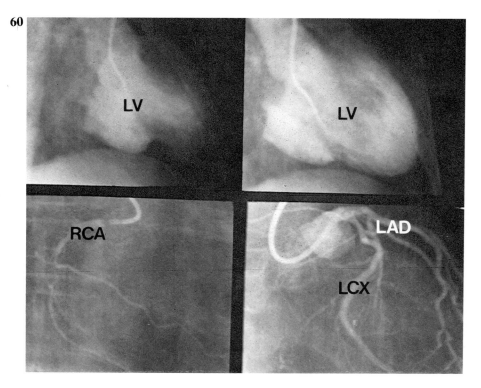

60 Inferior left ventricular aneurysm. Top left shows a systolic frame and top right shows a diastolic frame. The coronary arteriograms are shown below and it can be seen that the right coronary artery is blocked but the left coronary artery system is normal. LV–left ventricle; RCA–right coronary artery; LCX–left circumflex.

61 Pathology of a ruptured papillary muscle. A ruptured papillary muscle of the left ventricle of the heart in a patient who had had a myocardial infarction four days previously.

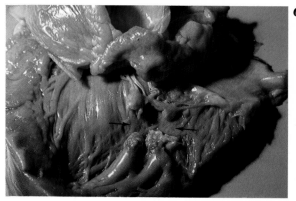

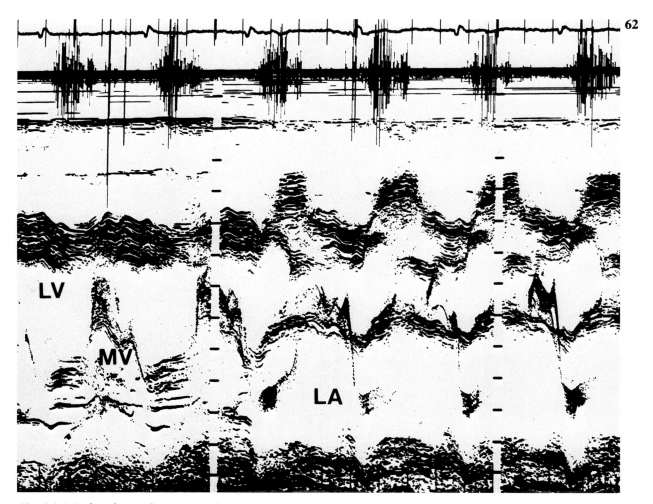

62 M- Mode echocardiogram with the mitral valve (MV) prolapsing into the left atrium (LA) in systole in a patient with a ruptured papillary muscle secondary to myocardial infarction. LV–left ventricle.

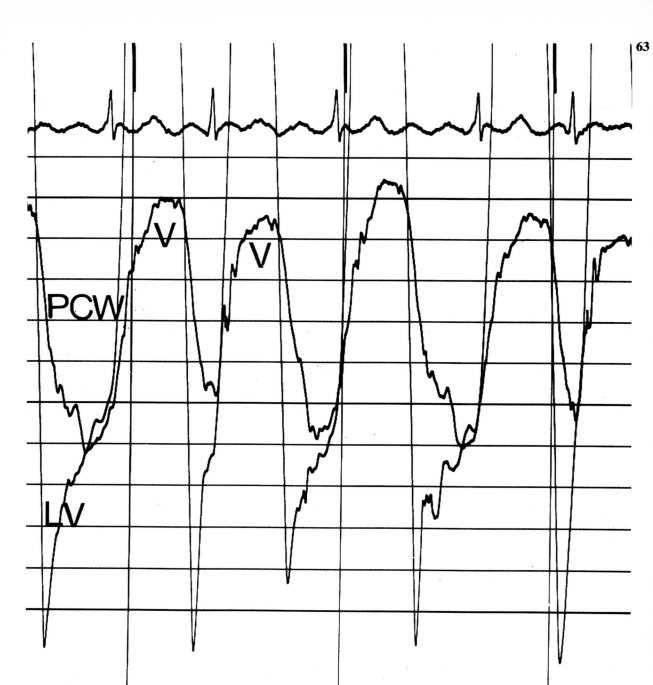

63   Pressure tracing taken at cardiac catheterisation with a left ventricular end-diastolic pressure (LV) and a simultaneous pulmonary capillary wedge pressure (PCW). A very dominant and tall V wave is seen on the pulmonary capillary wedge pressure tracing indicative of severe mitral regurgitation.

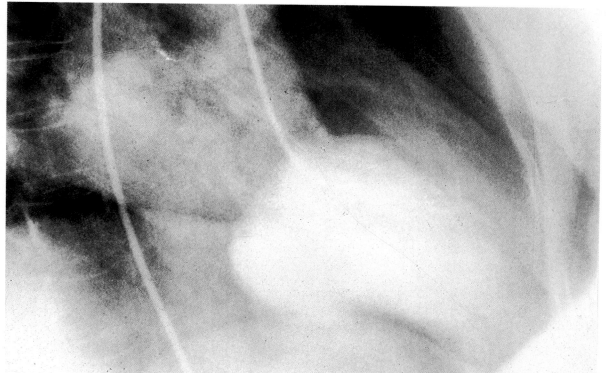

64 Left ventricular angiogram in a patient with a ruptured papillary muscle secondary to myocardial infarction. There is gross mitral regurgitation.

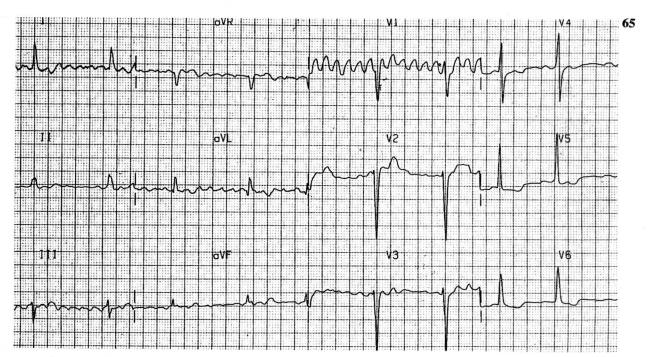

65 Electrocardiogram in which there is extensive Q wave changes in a patient who has poor left ventricular function due to previous myocardial infarction.

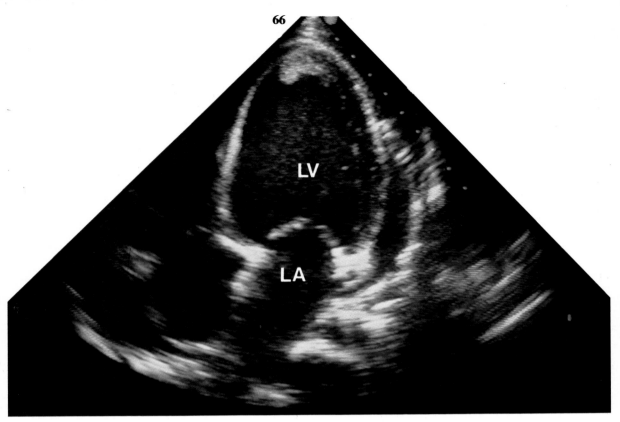

66 Two dimensional echocardiogram in a four chamber view in a patient with extensive ischaemic damage to the myocardium. The left ventricle (LV) is dilated and apical clot can be seen. LA–left atrium.

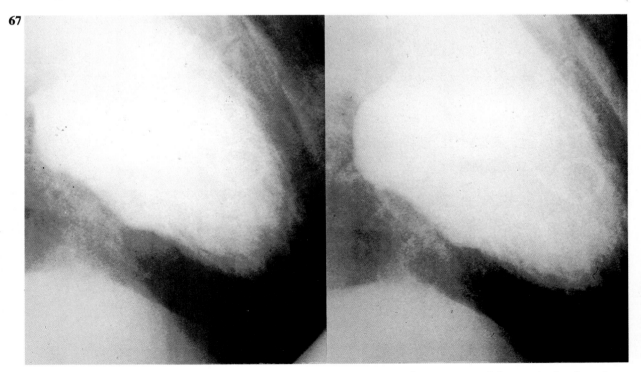

67 Left ventricular angiogram in systole (left) and diastole (right) showing poor left ventricular function in a patient with extensive myocardial damage due to ischaemic heart disease.

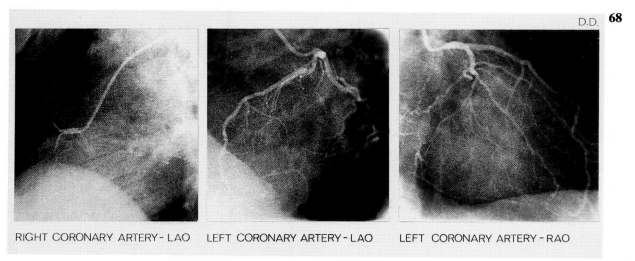

| RIGHT CORONARY ARTERY - LAO | LEFT CORONARY ARTERY - LAO | LEFT CORONARY ARTERY - RAO |

68 Coronary arteriogram in the same patient as in **65–67**, pages 105–106 in which there are multiple coronary lesions. LAO–left anterior oblique; RAO–right anterior oblique.

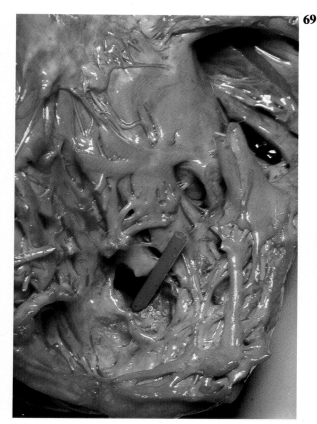

69

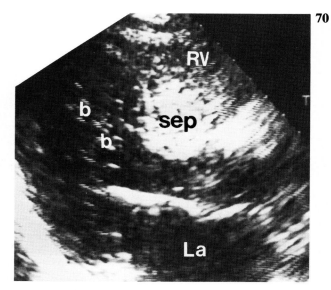

70

69 Pathology of ruptured interventricular septum. A ragged perforation is indicated by a blue rod in the lower part of the interventricular septum.

70 Two dimensional long axis parasternal echocardiogram; contrast study in a patient with ventricular septal defect after myocardial infarction. Contrast bubbles (b) can be seen in the left ventricle due to shunting from right ventricle (RV) to left. The left atrium (La) is free from contrast. sep-septum.

HEART FAILURE

1 Electron-microscopy of the myocardium in heart failure. The fibres are in disarray. There is ventricular hypertrophy as shown by the increased number of mitochondria.

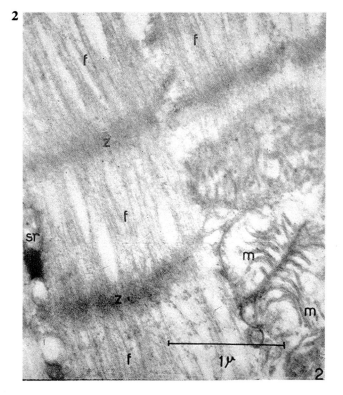

2 Electron-microscopy of the myocardium in heart failure. The mitochondria are shown to be swollen and there are also degenerative changes. SR—sarcoplasmic reticulum; F—myofibril; Z—z bands; M—mitochondria.

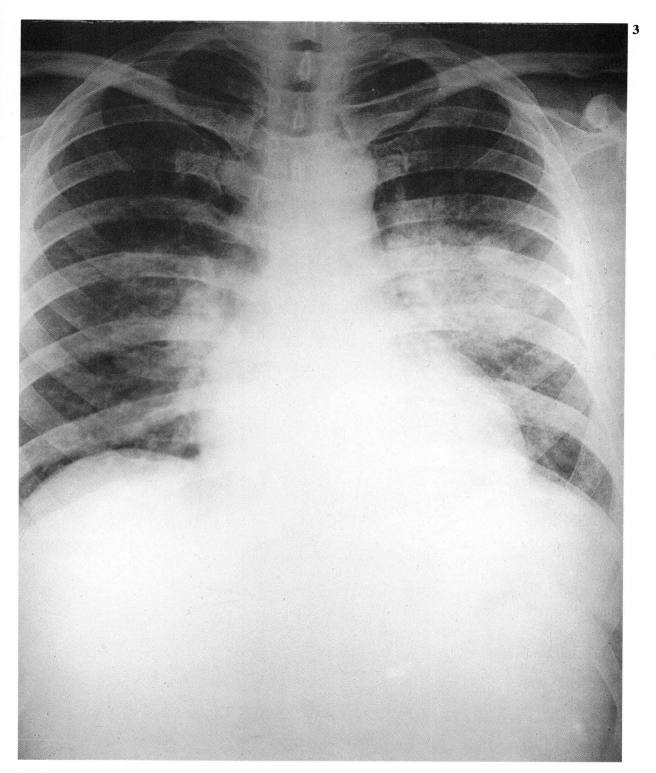

3 Chest x-ray showing a normal sized heart with severe pulmonary oedema in a patient with hypertensive heart failure.

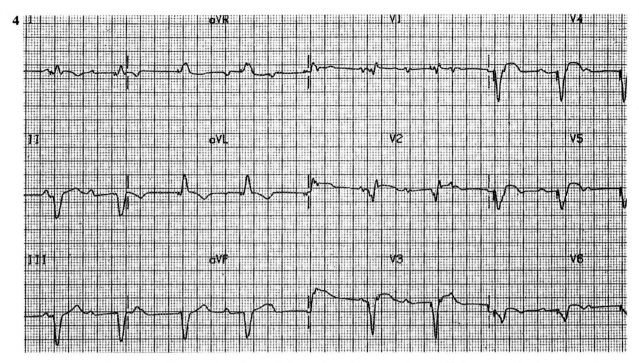

4 Electrocardiogram in hypertensive heart failure often shows evidence of left ventricular hypertrophy on voltage criteria with ST/T wave changes and frequently the rhythm is atrial fibrillation or atrial flutter.

5 Gated blood pool scan showing generalised and poor left ventricular function following the injection of technetium labelled red cells. The left ventricular function is severely impaired as evidenced by the absence of change in wall motion throughout the cardiac cycle.

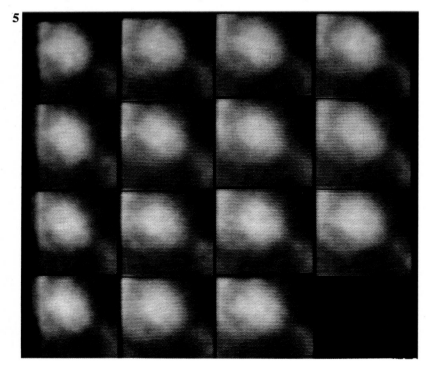

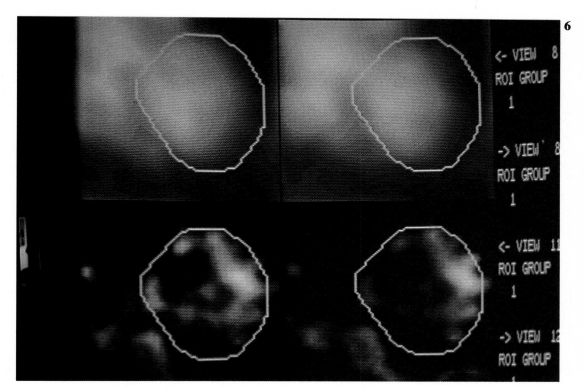

6 Gated blood pool scan. Computer superimposed systolic and diastolic frames; systole on the left and diastole on the right. The left ventricle is enclosed by the white line (the region of interest). Again it can be seen that there is generalised poor left ventricular function.

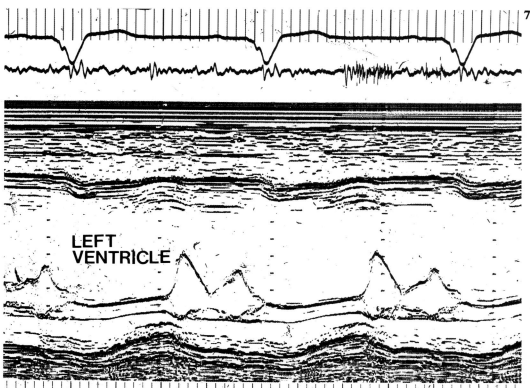

7

LEFT
VENTRICLE

7 M-Mode echocardiogram in a hypertensive patient with heart failure showing an enlarged cavity with reduced contraction.

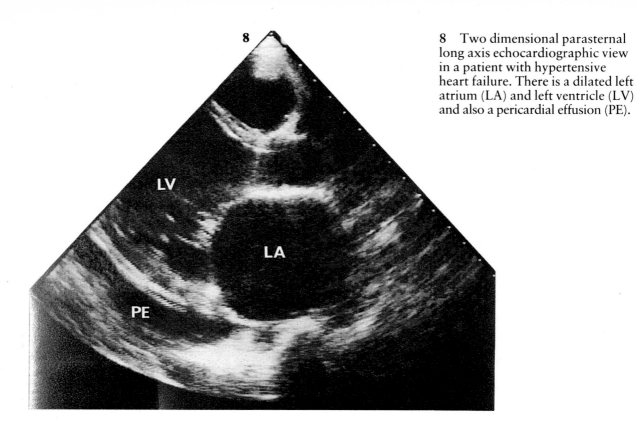

8 Two dimensional parasternal long axis echocardiographic view in a patient with hypertensive heart failure. There is a dilated left atrium (LA) and left ventricle (LV) and also a pericardial effusion (PE).

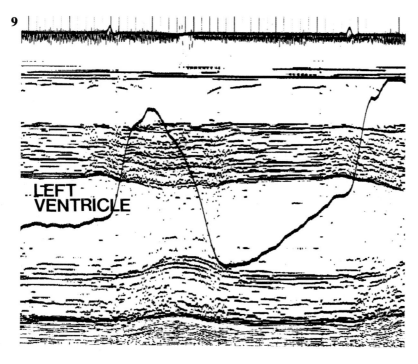

9 M-Mode echocardiogram in a patient with hypertensive heart failure. It can be seen that there is gross left ventricular hypertrophy, but there is no dilatation of the left ventricle.

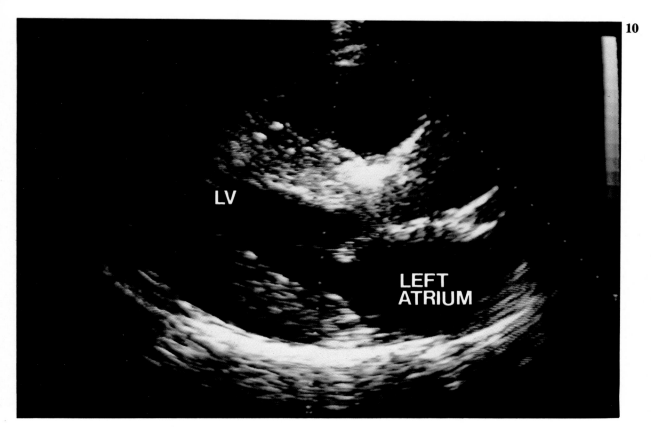

10 Two dimensional parasternal long axis echocardiographic view of a patient with hypertensive heart failure in which it can be seen again that there is severe left ventricular (LV) hypertrophy but there is no dilatation of the left ventricle.

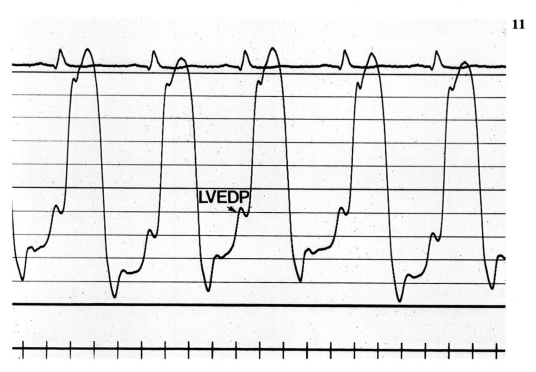

11 Pressure tracing recorded from a patient with hypertensive heart failure. The left ventricular end-diastolic pressure (LVEDP) is markedly elevated at 40 mmHg.

PERIPHERAL VASCULAR DISEASE

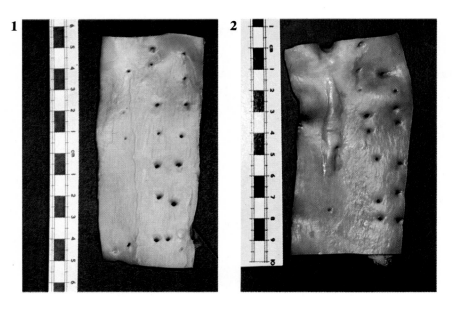

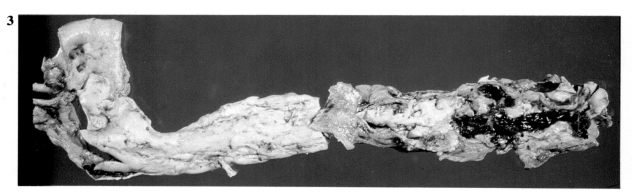

1   Pathology of atheroma. Extensive fatty streaking of the thoracic aorta in a young man. Apart from the left edge, most of the vessel is involved.

2   Pathology of atheroma. An elevated fibrous plaque in the thoracic aorta from a young man.

3   Pathology of atheroma. Ulcerated complicated lesions of advanced atherosclerosis in the aorta.

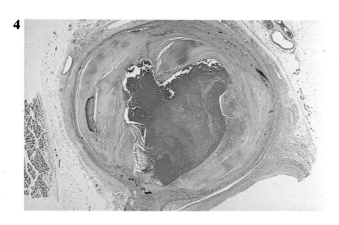

4   Histology of atheroma with recent thrombo-occlusion. Circumferential thickening of intima, patchy calcification of the plaques and marked atrophy of the media of this femoral artery, from a patient with gangrene of the left foot and leg. The lumen is filled with recent thrombus into which atheromatous debris including sterol clefts are present (H and E × 3).

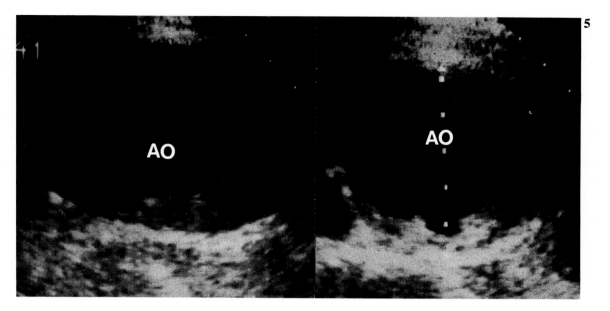

Longitudinal   Transverse

5   Longitudinal and transverse ultrasound sections through an abdominal aortic (Ao) aneurysm. The aneurysm measures more than 4 cm.

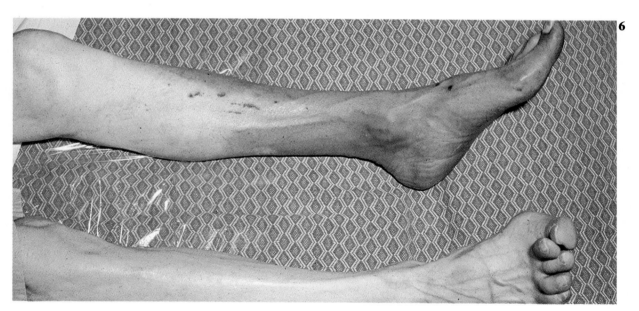

6   An ischaemic foot. Acute gangrene due to thrombo-occlusion of an atheromatous popliteal artery.

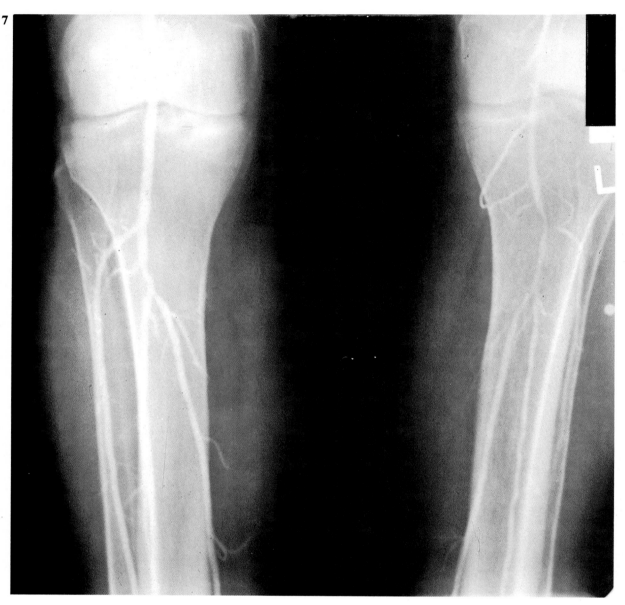

7 Peripheral phase of aortogram demonstrating severe atheromatous narrowing in the popliteal and tibial arteries of the left leg.

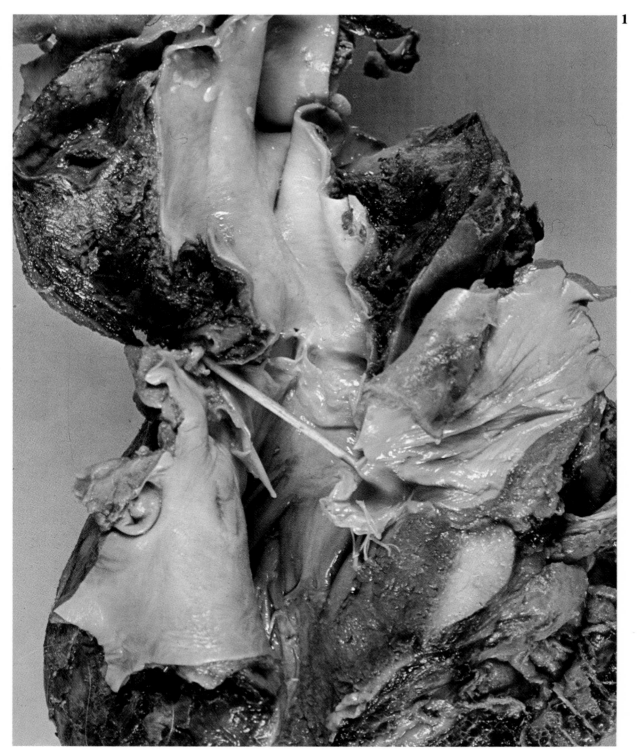

1   Pathological specimen of aortic dissection. The same patient is demonstrated in 2 and 3, pages 118 and 119. The aorta is dilated and surrounded by a large haematoma in the false lumen. The intimal flap is marked.

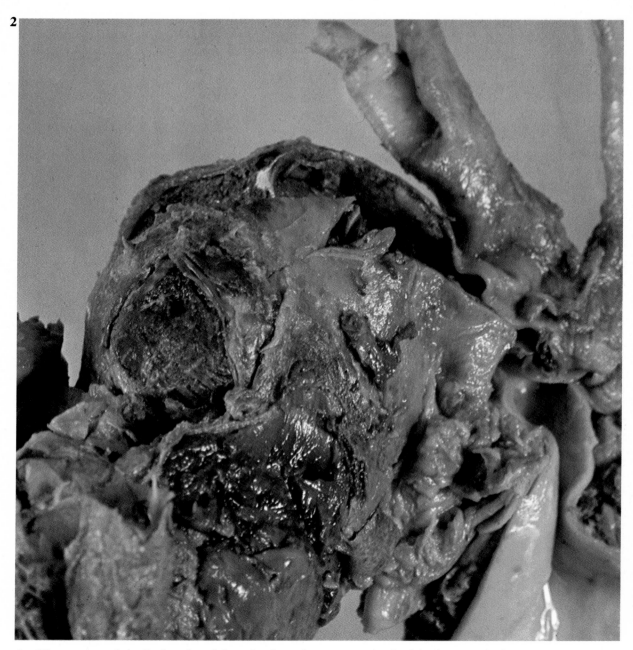

2 The aortic arch is displaced and there is a large haematoma in the false lumen which compresses the origin of the major arteries.

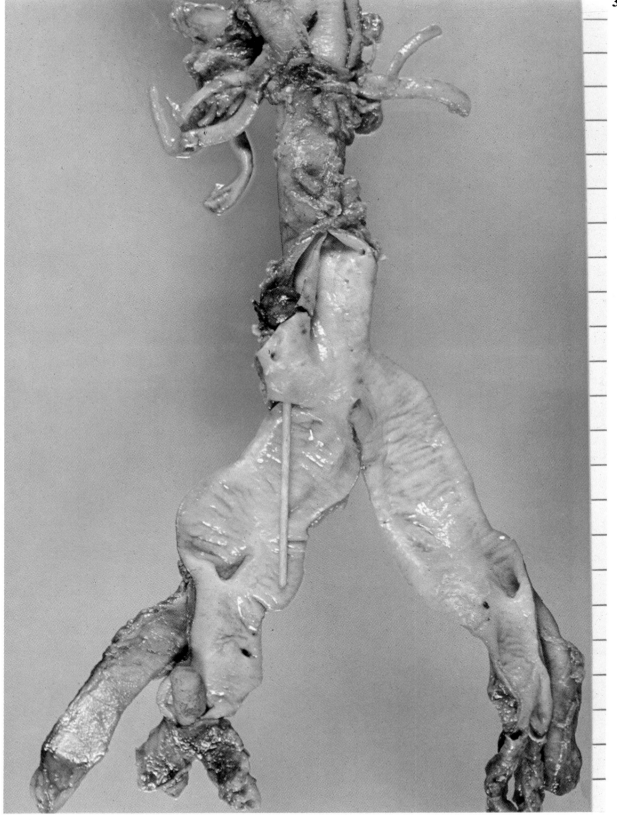

3   The point of re-entry of the dissection into the femoral artery is demonstrated by the marker.

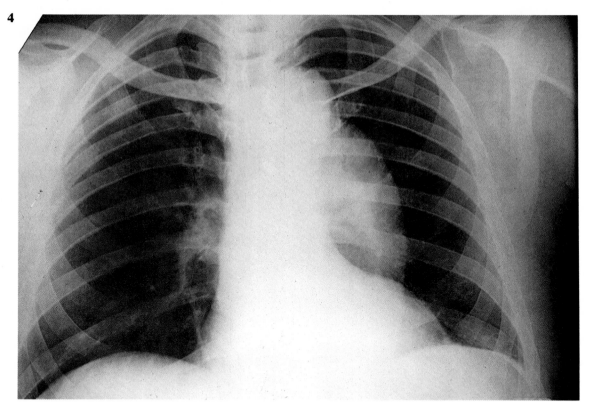

4 Chest x-ray of aortic dissection. Initially, hypertensive patients will show aortic dilatation which can be seen in the chest x-ray.

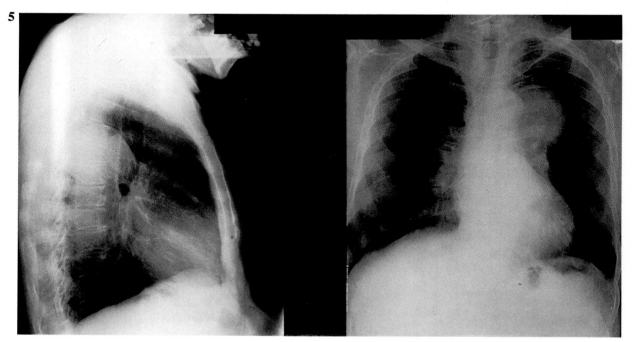

5 Chest x-ray with increasing aortic dilatation. An aortic aneurysm may develop and be seen as a posterior mediastinal mass.

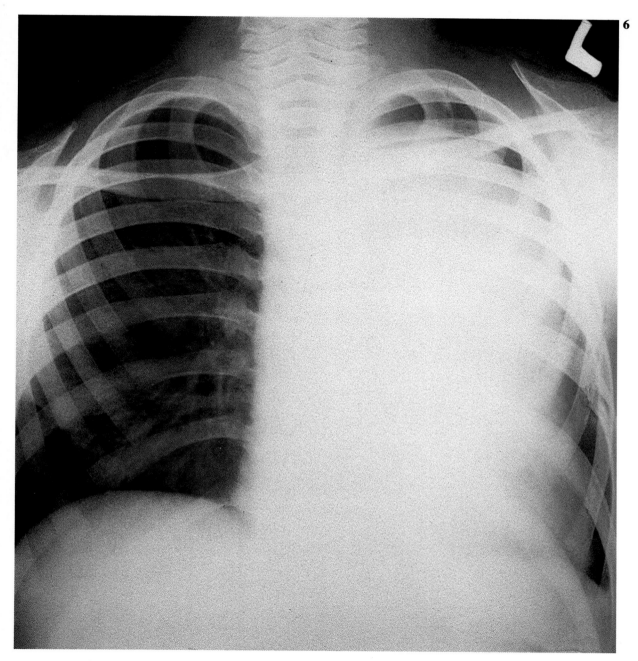

6 Extreme dilatation with dissection such that the aorta occupies almost the whole of the left hemithorax.

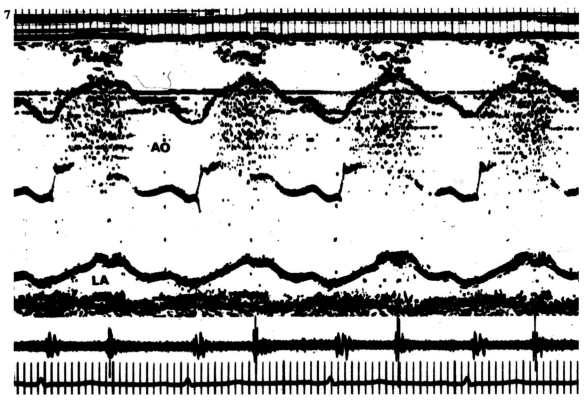

7 M-Mode echocardiogram. Hypertensive patient with a markedly dilated aortic root. However the motion of the aortic valve is normal. Ao–aortic; LA–left atrium.

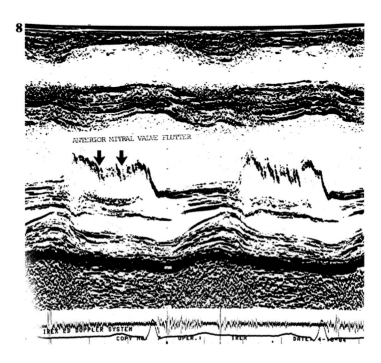

8 M-Mode echocardiogram. An enlarged left ventricle and mitral valve flutter due to severe aortic regurgitation that developed as a consequence of aortic dilatation and dissection.

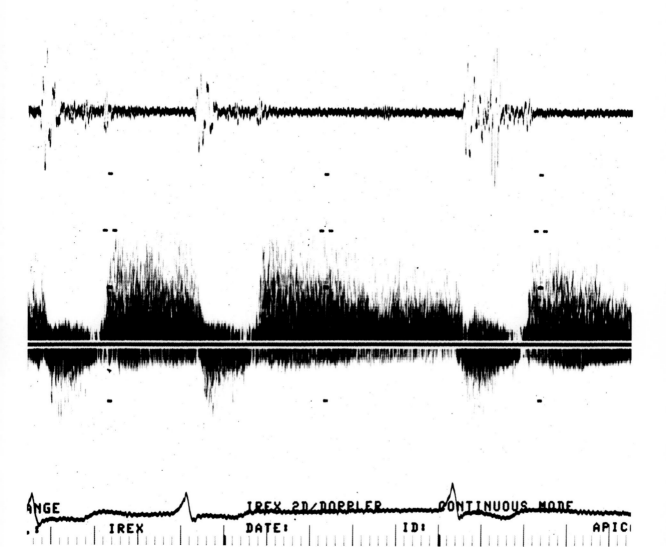

9 An apical continuous wave doppler study in the patient shown in 8, page 122. Blood flow below the baseline is away from the transducer and represents blood ejected into the aorta. Blood flow towards the transducer represents aortic regurgitation.

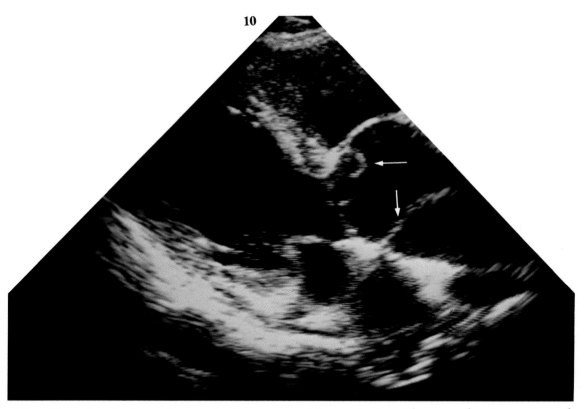

10 Two dimensional echocardiogram in the parasternal long axis view. This was taken in a patient who had hypertension and developed aortic dissection. The flap of the dissection may be seen both anteriorly and posteriorly (arrowed) and there is a huge aortic root.

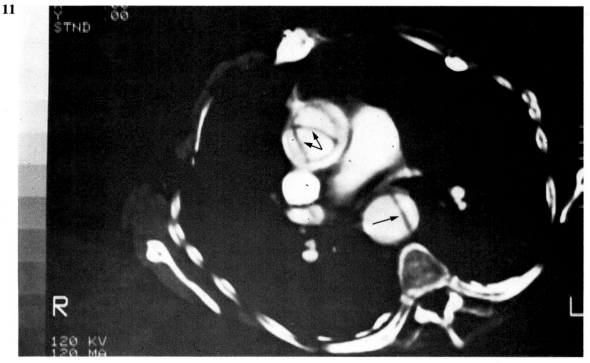

11 CT scan of aortic dissection in a patient with hypertension. The flaps (arrowed) can be seen both in the ascending and descending aorta.

12 A dilated aorta in a patient with hypertension. There is enlongation and folding of the aorta to produce a pseudo coarctation.

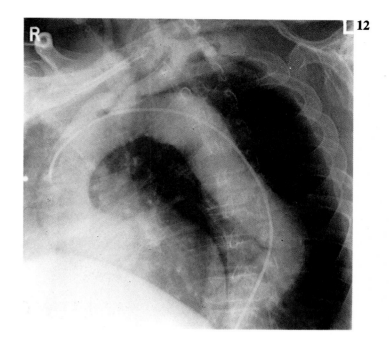

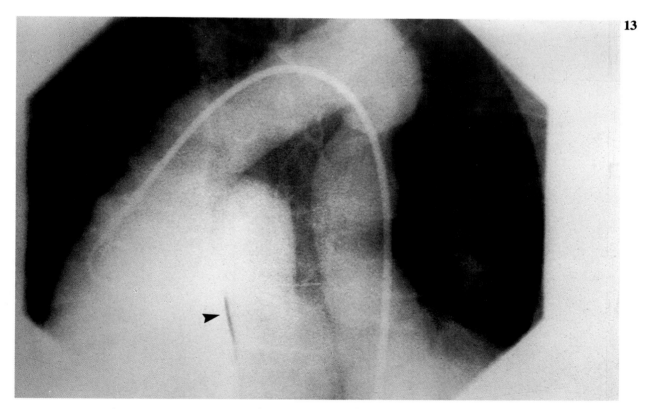

13 Aortogram showing an injection into the anterior saccular dilatation of an aortic dissection (arrowed).

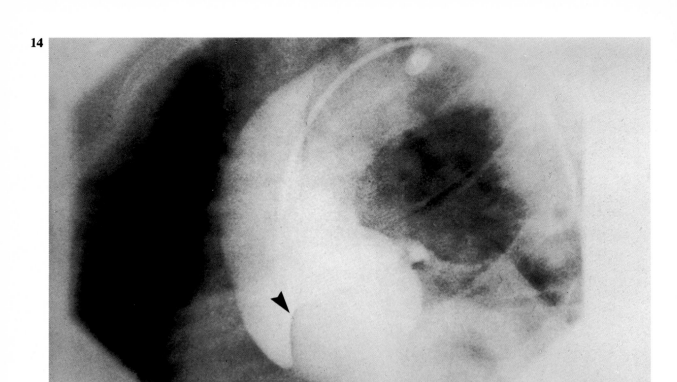

14 Aortogram. The origin of the aortic flap (arrowed) may be seen anteriorly and aortic regurgitation noted.

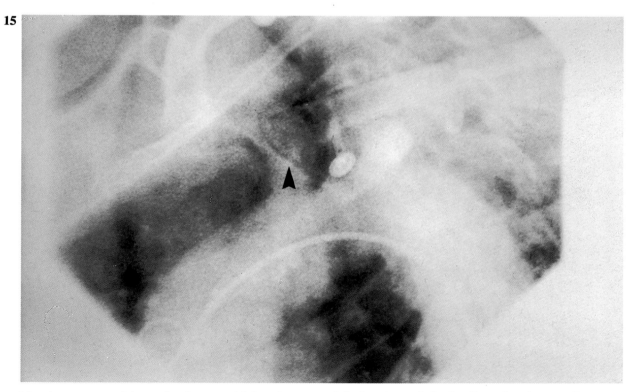

15 Aortogram of the arch of aorta with involvement of the head vessels in the dissection (arrowed).

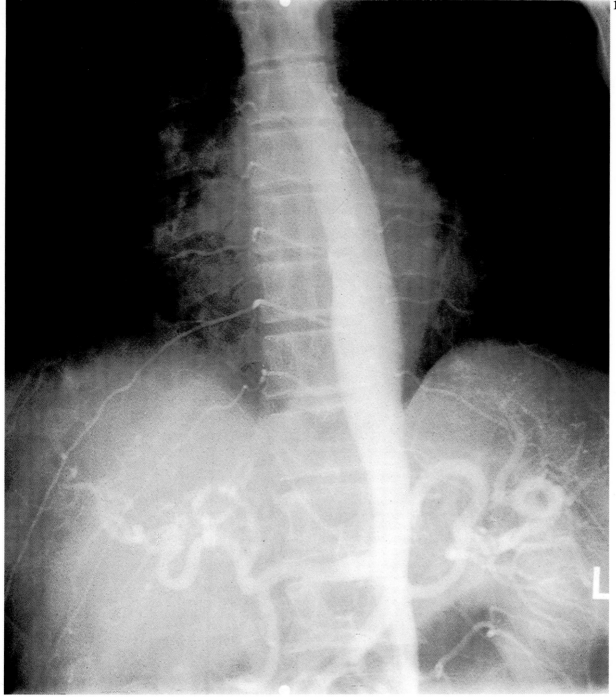

16 Aortogram showing the dissection flap extending down the descending aorta below the renal arteries.

KIDNEY

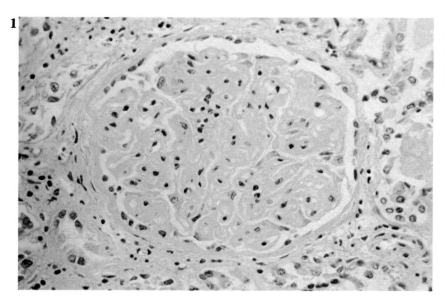

1 Histological section from a kidney with increased basement membrane thickening and pericapsular fibrosis due to hypertension (H and E × 512).

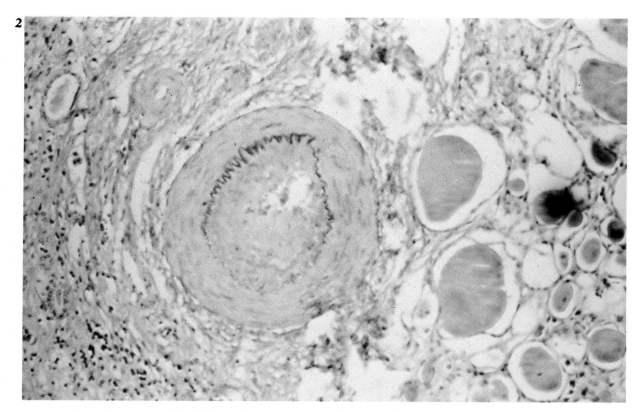

2 Histological section of the kidney showing arteriosclerosis with concentric thickening of the arteriolar wall.

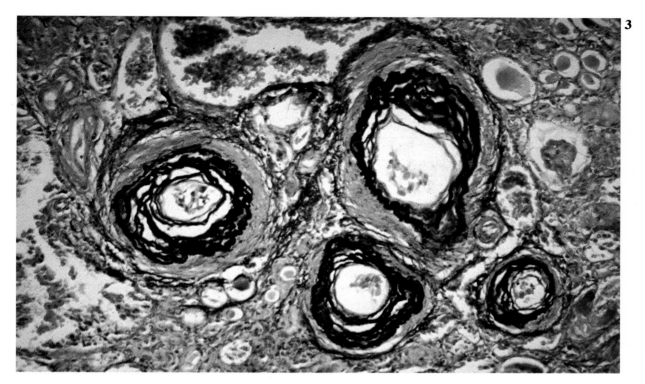

3 Histological section demonstrating the onion skin appearance of the arteriole with arteriolar obliteration (Elastic Van Gieson's stain).

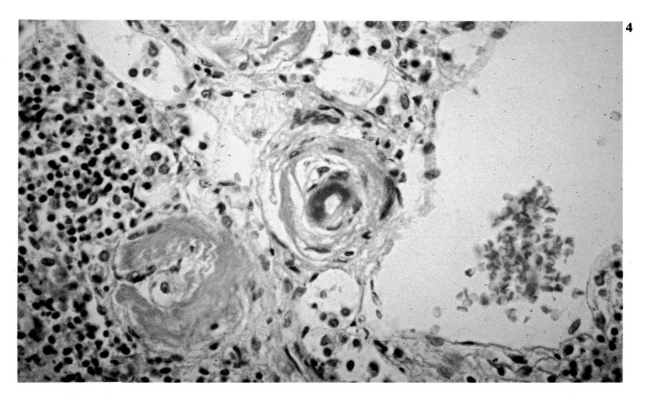

4 Histological section showing severe parenchymal changes resulting from arteriolar occlusion in the kidney.

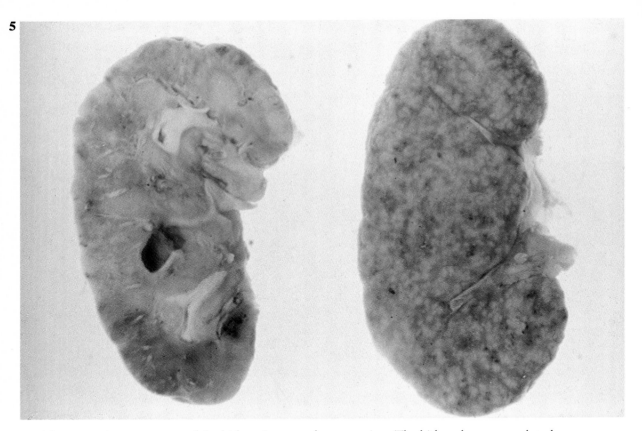

5 Macroscopic appearance of the kidney in severe hypertension. The kidney has a granulated appearance with numerous superficial haemorrhages.

BRAIN

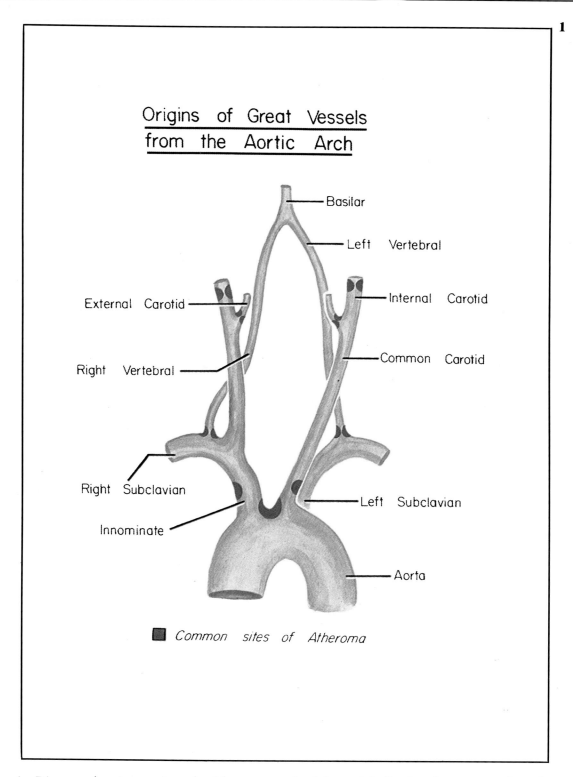

Origins of Great Vessels from the Aortic Arch

■ Common sites of Atheroma

1 Diagram showing aortic arch with great vessels of the neck indicating the common sites of atherosclerosis.

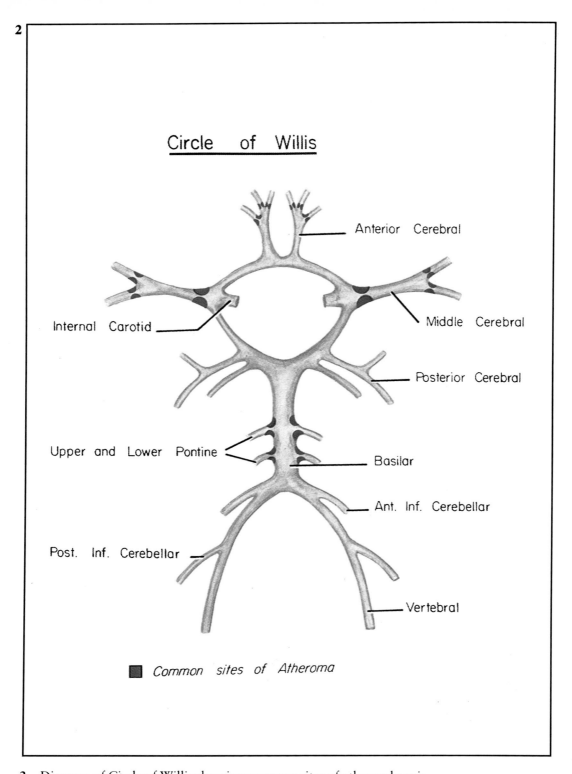

2 Diagram of Circle of Willis showing common sites of atherosclerosis.

3 Atheroma and occlusion of the internal carotid artery. The lumen of the left artery (right of picture) is reduced to a pinhole by atheroma. The right artery is occluded by a thrombus. There is severe atheroma of the posterior communicating and basilar arteries with irregularity of their walls (× 2.75).

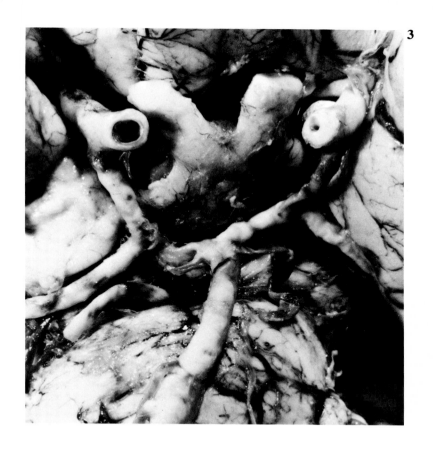

4 Normal carotid angiogram to be compared with **5**.

5 Carotid angiogram showing the common carotid and its bifurcation into the internal and external with a block of the internal carotid artery.

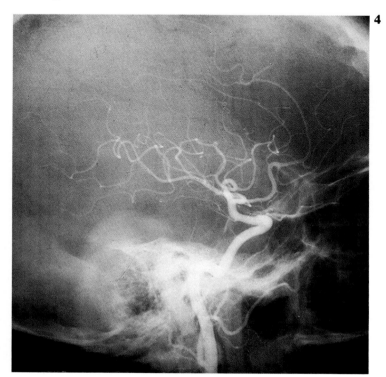

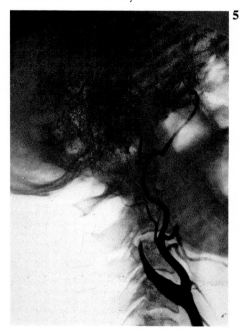

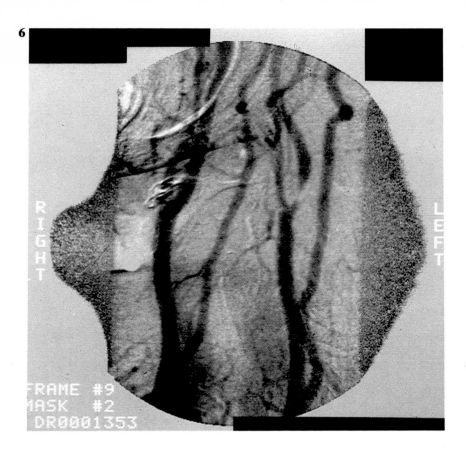

6 Digital subtraction angiogram showing significant stricture due to atheroma in the left internal carotid.

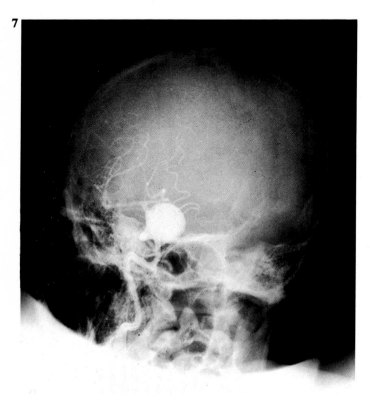

7 Carotid arteriogram showing a large carotid aneurysm.

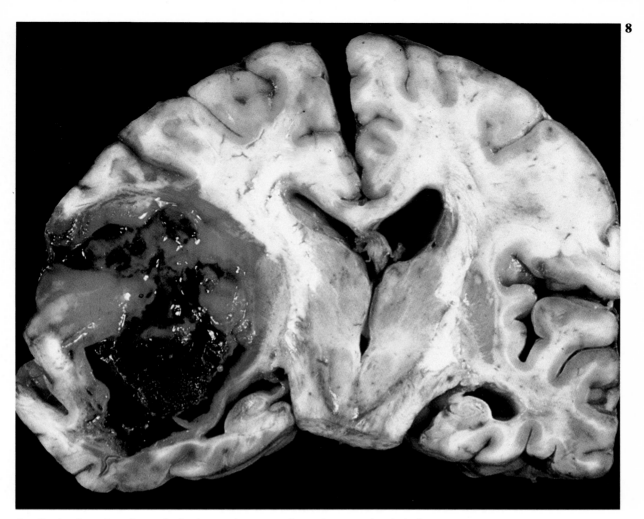

8   Sagittal section through the brain showing a large haemorrhagic infarct.

9

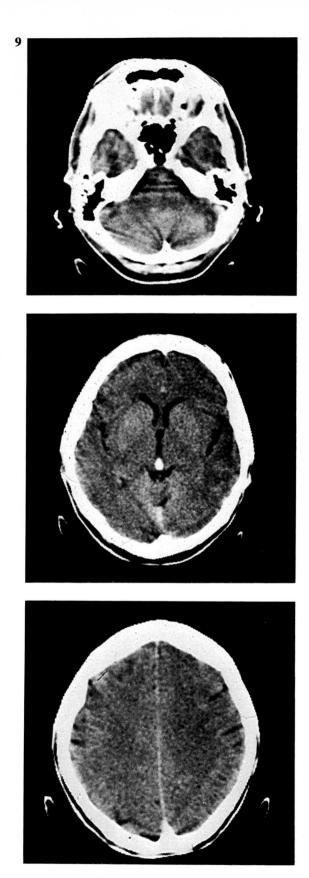

9   Normal CT scan to be compared with 10.

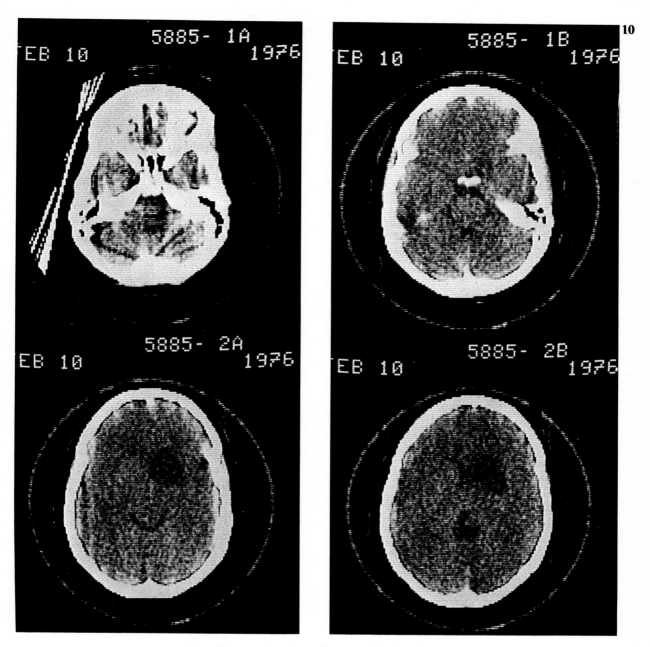

10 CT scan showing a large cerebral infarct.

Index

Index